Tony Cole

WHOSE
WELFARE?

Tavistock Publications · London · New York

First published in 1986 by
Tavistock Publications Ltd
11 New Fetter Lane,
London EC4P 4EE

© 1986 Tony Cole

Set by Hope Services, Abingdon
Printed in Great Britain by
Richard Clay (The Chaucer Press)
Bungay, Suffolk

*British Library Cataloguing
in Publication Data*

Cole, Tony
Whose welfare? – (Society now) –
(Social science paperback)
1. Welfare state – History
I. Title   II. Series
361.5′09   HN16

ISBN 0–422–60220–5

For my parents. Special thanks to Gerison for constant advice and support; to my daughter, Francine, who was born as I started the book and who provided regular inspiration and glorious interruptions; to Gill, whose typing was always efficient and accurate, and to the helpful staff of my college library at Loughton College of Further Education.

Contents

1

Introduction

What is social welfare?

Social welfare can be seen as the way societies meet the needs of their members. What, therefore, are people's needs? Very briefly, we can point to physical or biological needs as well as social or cultural ones. Whilst food is an obvious example of a biological need, it is also bound up with cultural needs as well; certain foods, for example, are laid down by custom, religion, and ritual.

In some societies the need for food is everyone's main lifelong preoccupation and is met through hunting, gathering, or fishing. These activities are not purely concerned with physical needs however. Being organized on a social basis and surrounded by beliefs and customs, they also serve to meet or express the cultural needs of their participants. In these societies there will be no separate social policy in the planned and deliberate sense; rather needs are met through traditional rules and customs. We have to remember, of course, that, in

1

any society, many needs go unmet or are met at the expense of other members of society.

In industrial societies very few people produce their own food. Food is a commodity to be bought and sold for money, as are many other needs. If we look, however, at the social distribution of money, it is clear that it is not just based on need. Inherited wealth, for example, gives wealth according to parentage rather than need.

Social policy and the problem of poverty

In societies largely based on the use of money to meet many of the members' needs and where the majority obtain their money by working, the situation of those with no work or who work for an inadequate income is often seen as a social problem. Social policy is the deliberate attempt to devise means to deal with social problems; the term, 'social policy', also refers to the academic subject which studies such policies.

The focus of this book is on policies, especially state policies, to deal with the problem of those on no or low income – that is, the problem of poverty. We should note, however, that the subject of social policy usually recognises five official welfare delivery systems: social security, health, education, housing, and the personal social services. Many commentators also refer to the way public transport, town planning, and economic policies can likewise affect people's welfare needs.

One of the main distinctions between the subjects of social policy and sociology is in their different approaches to social problems, such as that of poverty. Whereas social policy tends to focus on formulating, describing, or criticizing policies to solve the problem, sociology takes a quite different approach.

Not only would sociologists raise questions about the definition, measurement, extent, and causes of poverty, but they could also ask how and why it came to be defined as a social problem. There is a big difference between people on low incomes defining their situation as a problem and outside agencies, such as the government, seeing it as a problem and attempting to do something about it. The reasons why governments see poverty as a problem are also important, partly because that will affect how they react to it. Thus, if poverty is seen as a problem because 'the poor' are seen as a threat to the social order, then governments may adopt punitive policies to deal with it. Poverty may also be a problem for the state if it means that workers are too weak or unfit to be efficient workers or soldiers. In short, seeing why poverty comes to be seen as a problem helps us explain the general nature and growth of welfare provision.

Further reading

For a discussion of a sociological approach to social problems, see Berger (1966), especially pages 43–51, and Butterworth and Weir (1972), pages 15–34.

Social policy and social security

In looking at the various ways social policy has emerged to deal with the problem of poverty, we shall focus on government action, especially as it has developed in Britain and America. Those state policies of income support are often called social security.

There are and have been many other forms of welfare provision for the poor. In the past, charity played a much more significant part in poor relief than today, reflecting of course the near complete absence of state provision. In nineteenth century Britain and elsewhere, workers organized their own benefit schemes through trade unions and friendly societies and such provision continues to exist, though its significance has been reduced by an expanded state sector.

More crucially, from today's perspective Titmuss in his

essay, The Social Division of Welfare (1958), has pointed out that state spending on the social security budget is by no means the only way that income support is distributed in modern societies. Firstly, he refers to the system of tax allowances that reduce a person's tax to take account of particular circumstances; for example, home buyers get tax relief on their mortgages. Secondly, he points to the massive growth of occupational or company welfare in the form of company pension schemes, sick pay, subsidized goods, and services.

Activities

1 See if you can discover tax allowances, other than mortgage interest relief, for which a person can claim reduced tax. In what ways, if at all, do you think these tax allowances promote social welfare in society? Check your ideas against the section on tax allowances on pages 62 to 65.
2 By asking people you know, try to discover the range of benefits some workers receive in addition to their wages and salaries. Can you link this to the kind of work they do?

The aims and organization of this book

As noted above, this book concentrates on state policies of income support and poor relief. In practice, many wider aspects of welfare and its context will inevitably be raised and, through this, it is hoped to show that the study of welfare should be a crucial feature of any sociological analysis of society. Thus, we shall see how the British social security system has often assumed that women should be the dependants of men and denied them benefits accordingly. We shall also examine the degree to which 'the welfare state' has reduced class inequalities and the extent to which governments act on behalf of all or only some of their citizens, including its ethnic minorities and youth.

It is not just how the study of welfare feeds into these debates about inequality that makes it an important socio-logical topic. Social welfare can be seen as an important topic in its own right. In Britain, for example, about 30 per cent of state spending is on social security (an estimated £40 billion in 1985/86) and this excludes the cost in lost revenue of a range of personal tax allowances. Millions of people's incomes stem wholly or partly from social security. This is not to say that sociologists accept the state's definition of all this spending as 'welfare'. Just as sociologists have taken a sceptical view of state education and explored the possible role of school in social control and keeping people in their places, so too have sociologists asked similar questions of state welfare provision. Some sociologists have argued that welfare is best seen as a means of buying off unrest or discontent rather than as an expression of any genuine concern for need. It can also reinforce privilege as well as reduce deprivation. Similarly, just as sociologists of education have investigated which groups benefit most from schooling, sociologists of welfare have asked who gains most from state welfare spending and taxation.

These and other issues are explored both historically and by the use of literature on other societies, primarily America. The text includes a factual and theoretical account of social security developments in those societies and an examination of the main theoretical and ideological perspectives on welfare that have emerged in the last twenty years. Finally, there is a brief section on the British government's proposals for the reform of social security from 1988 onwards.

2

The pre-history of welfare

Sociological pointers

This section looks at the origins of state welfare in Britain. Through this it introduces the following general points that sociologists make about welfare:

(i) Welfare is sometimes used with or instead of repression as a way of trying to achieve social order.

(ii) The kind of welfare provision made can be linked, at least partly, to the ideas and interests of the dominant groups in society.

(iii) Thus, the concept of welfare cannot be taken at face value and cannot simply be seen in terms of meeting the needs of the deprived.

Modernization and the state

For many centuries much of pre-modern Europe was organized on feudal lines. Under this system monarchs held all the land, which was parcelled out downwards to nobility and lords of the manor; peasants or serfs then had access to the use of some of this land. In return, loyalty and either military or agricultural service was demanded. In England, this system began to decline from the thirteenth century onwards, as relationships became based more on money, wages, and rent.

Within feudalism there was a tendency for power to drift outwards, either to barons and lords or to the towns which slowly began to develop. Generally, education and poor relief (mainly charity) were the province of the church, with the state concerned only with external threats, internal order, and the defence of the faith, rather than administration as such.

At this stage then, the state was very unlike the modern state. Today the state claims the exclusive right to use force in a given territorial area; in those days there were many private armies. Today's state is theoretically organized on impersonal bureaucratic lines with written rules limiting its authority and that of its officials. Then it was more a question of barons tied by oaths of allegiance to the crown, though often building up their own power at the monarch's expense. This approach to the state draws on the analysis of Weber: a Marxist approach would stress the role of the state in the dominance of one class over another.

Activity

As a quick, approximate guide to the activities of the modern British state, draw up a list of the main government departments and what you think they do. A reference book such as *Pears Cyclopaedia* could help you here. You could do the same for the local state (or council).

The coming of the Poor Law

In the pre-industrial era many European states began to

develop more centralized power structures. In England, the Tudor period was crucial in the development of the modern, centralized nation-state. Many writers have argued that the origins of Poor Law at this time reflected the Tudor state's anxiety about the threat to its development and security from the disorder arising from vagrancy and poverty. One writer states:

> 'It was undoubtedly fear of social disorder in the two and a half centuries following the Black Death which gradually converted the maintenance of the poor from an aspect of personal Christian charity into a prime function of the state.'

> (Fraser 1973)

Originally the Tudors sought to repress the vagrancy 'by police measures of hideous brutality' (Tawney 1936) but the rising numbers of poor and a growing recognition that it had economic and not simply personal causes began to change this. Though the able-bodied poor were still treated with great severity, in 1536 parishes were empowered to collect money for the impotent poor to save them from begging, establishing some small role for the state for those who cannot work. Even so private charity remained a bigger source of assistance for the poor, at least until the 1660s.

The ideology and practice of poor relief

Up until the sixteenth century then, relief for the poor (i.e. the majority of the population) was the preserve of charity organized through the church. The poor were seen to be God's friends, as were those who gave to the poor; the stewardship and paternal responsibility of the rich was stressed, though not always fulfilled. Thus the existence of poverty was justified as itself a state of grace and as a means by which the rich could elevate themselves by the act of giving. Such a neat justification of wealth and poverty illustates precisely Berger's statement that 'We speak of an

8

ideology when a certain idea serves a vested interest in society' (Berger 1966).

From the sixteenth century onwards, social change was beginning to bring new social groups and ideas to the fore. The increase in the importance of trade was giving rise to a merchant class, whose ideas and outlooks were called mercantilism. The Protestant Reformation and the growth of Puritanism, itself linked to the rise of the middle classes, was also to exert a major influence on social theory and social policy.

In Britain and France, mercantilism was associated with an emphasis on the trading strength of the nation and, though workers were seen with contempt, some concern for their welfare was necessary if they were to add to national economic well-being. Idleness (i.e. unemployment) was seen to discourage work habits and high wages were seen to encourage the worker's natural tendency to laziness, crudity and riotous behaviour! As a result, the question of work for the able-bodied poor was to become central to English Poor Law in the Elizabethan period and beyond; work was seen to be beneficial both to the nation's wealth and the worker's character.

The most important single measure of the whole Tudor, and indeed pre-industrial, period was the 1601 Act, known as the forty-third of Elizabeth. The Act was based on making clear-cut definitions of categories of poor and the ways they were to be dealt with. Those defined as the impotent poor (the aged, chronic sick, blind, lunatic) were to be provided with relief within institutions such as almshouses. The able-bodied poor were to be provided with work, outside initially, but later in workhouses; if they absconded they were to be sent to houses of correction. In addition to these measures, Justices of the Peace were given the responsibility of regulating wages, bread prices, and the quality of products.

Whilst the scheme was to be locally administered, its significance was that it was to be national in structure, with overall supervision by the Privy Council.

The decline of the Elizabethan Poor Law

Over the next two centuries, at least four major influences shaped the development of this policy:

(i) The failure to fully implement the Act. There were enormous variations in the speed and extent to which the provisions were applied in practice. The English Civil War (1640s) and other factors actually weakened the power of central government and local autonomy of Poor Law implementation increased. Additionally, separate institutions of care, work, and punishment were never built and the workhouse became a catch-all institution.

(ii) The system of economic regulation of wages and prices began to decline. As the amount of trade, commerce, and later industrial development grew, prices came to be governed increasingly by the forces of supply and demand – the market economy was emerging.

(iii) With the development of industrialization in England from the mid-eighteenth century onwards, enormous social changes began to occur, placing increased demand and costs on the system of poor relief. Many local initiatives were introduced to deal with this hardship and the bad harvests of the 1790s. The most notable derived from the Berkshire village of Speenhamland and involved giving subsidies to wages out of the rates, based on the price of bread and the size of the household in need.

(iv) The growth in the influence of Puritanism was mentioned earlier but now needs further discussion, not least because it was strongly linked with the rising commercial and, later, industrial bourgeoisie. The 1601 Act had encouraged private charity which had grown in the first four decades of the seventeenth century. From then on, however, it came under attack from Puritanism. The impact of this Protestantism was that those with success and wealth saw this as a sign of God's favour. Naturally, therefore, poverty was seen as a sign of personal deficiency and, indeed, a punishment for sin. Charity was condemned as undermining the work ethic. The basic tenet underlying this new world view was that of individual rather than social responsibility and thus the poor should be left to their own resources – or lack of them. The Poor Law was made stricter and more punitive with the threat of the workhouse increasingly used to deter people from claiming relief; beggars and vagrants were given a choice between forced labour and a whipping.

Whilst these harsh values were moderated by the mid-eighteenth century, they were revived in a different guise in the early nineteenth century. Philosophers, economists and others once again came to attack the paternalism, cost, and workings of the Poor Law system. These were the theorists of the new industrial order whose ideas more closely fitted the interests and outlooks of the industrial capitalists who were beginning to shape the world in their own image.

Further reading

For a useful but challenging discussion of the links between history and sociology, see Carr (1964), especially pages 47 and 65–7, or C. Wright Mills (1970), Chapter 8, especially pages 162–71.

An account of the possible connections between Puritanism, class, and the rise of capitalism, based on the work of Max Weber, can be found in most sociology textbooks.

3

1834: sociology and social welfare – origins and foundations

Introduction

It is possible to trace the origins of sociology and the foundations of modern welfare (in Britain, at least) to the early decades of the nineteenth century. Indeed, if we wanted to celebrate a birthday, Townsend (1981) has suggested that '1834 would be an appropriate year to begin any account of the foundations of British sociology'.

The general reason for the emergence of sociology at that time is rooted in the nature of the sociological perspective, briefly referred to earlier. As we have seen, Berger (1966) makes a distinction between how society might be seen by the powerful and how sociologists might understand it. Prior to the French Revolution (1789) and the Industrial Revolution in Britain, the forces of tradition, the authority of custom and religion, embedded in village life, and the enormous power of rulers restricted the development of alternative views of the world. Much of the sociology of the period, born of these social changes, was an attempt to explain their origins and explore their consequences.

The specific importance of 1834 derives from two related events of that year. Firstly, the publication of the Report of the Commission of the Poor Law set up in 1832, following the criticisms referred to briefly in Chapter One, and then the passing of the report's recommendations into law. Secondly, there was the setting up of the Statistical Society. The former was part of the social policy of the new ruling groups or elites to force the uprooted labouring classes to accept the disciplines of the emerging economic order: low wages, long hours, poor working conditions. The latter was representative of a growing concern with knowledge about and measurement of society: it can be seen as a necessary part of any concerted policy aimed at organizing society in a new way and managing its social problems. Out of this concern also came social surveys, commissions of inquiry and so on; these eventually led on to the development of the academic discipline of social policy/social administration, as well as shaping the early growth of sociology.

The new Poor Law

The old system under attack

In the introduction, we saw how sociologists and others have questioned the use of the term 'welfare' and indicated that it may be used to cover a wide range of intentions and effects. Some of the complexity of the concept is illustrated in the following criticisms made of the system of poor relief operating in England prior to the Poor Law Amendment Act, 1834:

(i) It was not adequate to the task of relieving or preventing poverty, especially after the massive changes brought about by industrialization, urbanization, and the rapid growth of population (from an estimated 9¼ million in 1781 to 16½ million in 1831).

(ii) Despite this failure, many ratepayers and commentators saw its cost as a burden; an estimated 10 per cent of the population were on relief in 1803 and, in 1815, an estimated 100,000 paupers were in workhouses.

(iii) To many of the propertied classes, this burden might have been tolerable if it had acted as effective insurance against unrest among the poor but it did not. In 1830 there were agricultural riots in areas covered by the Speenhamland system (see page 10).

(iv) Speenhamland itself and poor relief generally came under increasing theoretical or ideological attack. In particular, relief was said to demoralize the worker by undermining hard work and independence – the focus of this concern was nearly always on the able-bodied poor rather than the old, sick, or orphaned. These ideas are explored more later.

(v) Poor relief and labour mobility. The economist Adam Smith saw that the expanding industrial capitalism required that village labourers be prepared to move to the growing towns and factories. He argued that the 1662 Act of Settlement, empowering parishes to remove newcomers from the village if they appeared likely to become chargeable on the rates, prevented many people leaving their villages to seek work elsewhere. Modern historians believe these restrictions on labour mobility were probably over-estimated, but as Fraser notes on the 1834 Report, 'What people thought was happening was, for the purpose of social policy, more important than what was actually happening' (Fraser 1973).

Sociological note

It is worth noting here that this comment precisely illustrates the perspective of the early twentieth century American sociologist W. I. Thomas, who argued that once people define situations as real, they become real in their consequences. This idea became incorporated into the sociological perspective called symbolic interactionism. Interactionist theories emphasize the way people interpret and define their social world and act on these definitions. Whilst they have their problems, these theories are a counter to those sociologists and historians who write as if social action and social change were merely an automatic response to external forces and conditions. Such writers often see welfare development in terms of some inevitable force like 'progress'. This is discussed further on pages 28 and 46.

Social and ideological background

The largely rural, agricultural society of mid-eighteenth century England had, by 1830, become an increasingly urban, industrial one. This brought with it a major shift in the class structure.

Previously, it had been common for ordinary people to work for themselves on land they owned or rented and, at home, spinning or weaving, as an employee of someone else, who owned the yarn, cloth, and machinery – a capitalist. The dominant groups in this society were the landowners and gentry, though the church also had considerable power. These people generally owed their position to inheritance rather than achievement. Indeed their culture was one of leisure rather than work, and may have embodied a traditional, paternal concern for the poor.

As 1830 arrived, ordinary people were increasingly town dwellers who relied for their living solely on working for someone else, a millowner, for example. They were, in Marx's terminology, the proletariat. The nation's wealth was no longer predominantly based on land; rather it was derived increasingly from manufacturing and trade, giving wealth and power to its owners. Though some of these capitalists drew on 'old wealth', many had built up fortunes from comparatively humble origins and their outlooks reflected this. They stressed hard work, competition, and the individualist view that people can determine their own destinies; what has been called the entrepreneurial ideal or simply middle-class ideology. They saw economic success as a reward for positive personal qualities. Conversely, poverty was a sign of inadequacy, of failure to conform successfully to the dominant values just outlined. For this it was to be stigmatized and punished. Poor relief was seen as an encouragement to laziness, alcoholism, excessive fertility, fraud, and vice.

One theorist of such views was the Rev. Malthus who linked his attack on poor relief to a theory of population. Poor relief encouraged people to early marriage and parenthood regardless of their independence. It took resources from the productive and gave them to the unproductive and therefore made more people prone to pauperism. In short, poor relief undermined the morality of the poor and increased their numbers. Rimlinger (1971) has noted that, whilst the theory was of questionable validity, its view that the hardship of the poor and the wealth of the rich were equally justified made the theory appeal to the latter.

Not only were there firm beliefs about work and individualism but also about the workings of the economy and the proper role of government. Adam Smith had argued that the economy was self-regulating, guided by a hidden hand. Government interference in trade, industry, employment, or society generally was considered unnecessary and undesirable. This doctrine of minimal government was to influence social policy for the rest of the century, and beyond. Any attempts by the newly forming trade unions to improve wages or working conditions were similarly opposed as meddling with market forces, as interfering in the supposedly freely negotiated contract of employment between the individual worker, possibly ten years of age, and his or her employer. Trade unions were outlawed in 1799 and 1800 and continued to face legal restrictions even after these Acts were repealed in 1824.

Whilst Malthus and his followers opposed any poor relief, the 1834 Report accepted relief for the weak, sick, and elderly and even for the able-bodied poor so long as it was under harsh and punitive conditions. This report represented the triumph of the new liberalism (laissez-faire individualism) over traditional paternalism.

16

The Poor Law Amendment Act, 1834 – agenda and proposals

In the shaping of social policy and the exercise of power generally, it is important to look at what is called agenda setting, a process which 'presents a limited range of policy options as inevitable, probable or impracticable, very much according to the current wisdom in the corridors of state' (Golding and Middleton 1982). The 1834 Report set the agenda by omitting or understating the following issues:

(i) It underplayed the influence squalid housing, poor sanitation, and dirty, dangerous working conditions could have on working-class life.

(ii) It dealt only minimally with poverty among the elderly, orphaned, and sick.

(iii) It assumed unemployment among the able-bodied was self-chosen and wilful rather than related to such structural factors as lack of work and economic upheaval.

The Act itself was based on three key principles:

(i) The Poor Law should be run by a central authority. This proposal seems to run counter to the doctrine of laissez-faire. It was consistent, however, with another view strongly held by the Report's authors. This was a firm and optimistic belief that the new 'scientific study of society' could be rationally applied to problem solving and that bureaucratic organization was the most efficient means of pursuing this.

(ii) Relief was to be made conditional on entry into a workhouse which would 'moralize' the pauper. Paupers were those with no livelihood and who relied on relief or begging. They were categorized as moral defectives and seen as quite distinct from the poor on low incomes.

(iii) Conditions in the workhouse were to be set at a level lower than any likely to be met outside. This so-called principle of less eligibility was designed to ensure that even the lowest wages available were more attractive than the workhouse.

The historian E. P. Thompson (1968) quotes one administrator of a Norfolk workhouse as recording that his policy of reducing inmates' diets had been less effective as a deterrent to workhouse entry than ' "a minute and regular observance of routine", religious exercises, silence during meals, "prompt obedience", total separation of the sexes, separation of families, labour and total confinement'. He also forbade paupers from keeping their own possessions such as clothing or soap and noted, with satisfaction, how his policy led twelve women paupers to leave the workhouse.

In short, the Act was designed to deter paupers rather than relieve the poor.

Activities and further reading

1 Using either Goffman's own book, *Asylums* (1968), or an account of his work in a textbook, look up his analysis of mental hospitals and other total institutions. (These are combined places of work and residence, such as prisons or boarding schools.) Look at what Goffman sees as the central characteristics of these institutions and how they are organized to 'change' the inmates but often do so in unintended ways. Compare this with the brief outline of workhouse organization given above.

2 For those interested in more historical background, Dickens's *Oliver Twist* gives a good fictional account of workhouse life, from a very critical perspective.

The American experience

Sociologists sometimes seek to further their understanding of an issue by comparing different societies. Here, observation of American arguments over poor relief present interesting differences from and similarities with England. Much of this discussion is drawn from Rimlinger's work in this field (1971).

America and, to a lesser extent, Canada have been welfare

laggards compared to Western Europe. Even today they rank low in international comparisons of spending on income maintenance (Kudrle and Marmor 1981). The laggard status of the US can be linked to the following factors, stressing influences of class, immigration, culture and ideology:

(i) Firstly, there are significant differences between the development of US society and that of European society. Notable here is the absence of a feudal past with its connotations of paternalism. Consequently, America had no tradition of protection of the poor by the rich, however inadequate this might have been in practice. As a result there was less opposition in higher circles to the doctrine of laissez-faire individualism than there was in England and, especially, Germany.

(ii) Secondly, there is the direct question of America's colonial and immigrant background. Initially, the American colonies had taken over the English relief scheme but the newly independent nation was strongly against it. The Americans noted that many paupers were recent immigrants, sometimes direct from the English workhouse. To an extent, pauperism was seen as an alien disease, a failure of newcomers to adapt to the new society and capitalize on its supposedly unlimited opportunities.

It has been suggested that Canada's slightly earlier welfare development can be partly explained by the presence there, among English immigrants, of both socialist values and old-fashioned upper-class Tory paternalism. The other major immigrant group came from France, many of whom had left France before the libertarian, anti-state authority ideals of the French Revolution had had a chance to influence them significantly.

(iii) The third factor also relates to the question of immigration and concerns the American class structure. Compared to its employed working class, nineteenth century America had a large self-employed, independent producer class. Thus factory workers in the East, often immigrants, had the prospect of moving into self-employment, preventing the development of a stable, hereditary working class. Where this prospect was a myth, the 'American Dream' was still powerful enough to offer the hope of such and thus prevent the development of class consciousness on European lines. For example, trade unionism was limited and working-class socialism almost non-existent. The working class was also divided on national, religious, and regional lines and there was the massive barrier to class solidarity presented by widespread racism to the large (ex-) slave black population.

(iv) Finally, we must note the powerful influence of the ideology of liberalism in American dominant circles. This was strongest in the decades after their Civil War (1861–65). Immigration and urbanization proceeded rapidly, bringing major social problems. The response was a concerted defence of laissez-faire. The hostility to poor relief was given theoretical support by the English sociologist Herbert Spencer, who toured America and was treated to lavish banquets by wealthy businessmen. He drew on the evolutionary theories of Darwin, which were already gaining acceptance among American scientists, and applied them to the development of society. This social Darwinism argued that social progress came through competition and the survival of the fittest; poor relief therefore was seen as interfering with the natural laws of progress and purification. The poverty, sickness, and death of the weak or orphaned were all seen as necessary to the ultimate higher good. His ideas were adopted and adapted by the American sociologist Sumner, who asserted that 'the millionaires are a product of natural selection, acting . . . to pick out those who can meet the requirements of certain work to be done' (quoted in Rimlinger 1971), whereas the poor included 'the negligent, shiftless, inefficient, silly, and imprudent . . . the idle, intemperate and vicious'.

These and other writers reinforced a deeply held hostility to any but the smallest state intervention.

Women, work, and welfare in Victorian Britain – the rise of the family wage

So far, like much history and sociology, the writing has referred to social classes or the poor but has not differentiated on grounds of gender. This must be remedied. Not only was (and is) there inequality between women and men in society but social policy has often reflected and reinforced this. It has, to some extent, been the work of feminists in these areas to 're-discover' some of the processes by which this inequality was produced and is sustained. In doing this, they have shown how these academic disciplines have often reflected the dominant male assumptions of wider society.

Earlier we saw how the industrial revolution made waged work outside the home the main or only source of household income and, with this, labour at home ('housework') lost touch with the public world of money, status and recognition (Himmelweit 1983). Initially, men were a minority of waged workers but gradually this changed as middle-class reformers campaigned against child and female labour on 'protective' grounds. Sometimes this reforming spirit came from a Puritanical zeal which looked on the mines, for example, as 'indecent' places for women to work. Women's role in providing a moral environment at home came to be increasingly stressed and they came to be defined primarily as wives and mothers. These roles had assumptions of nurturance and dependency.

In addition to these reforming pressures, male-dominated working-class organizations sought to strengthen their position by reducing the supply of labour, that is excluding women and children. They could also then argue for the need for a higher wage to support a family. Thus was born the ideology of the family wage, the idea that there should be one wage earner per family and that he, for it was assumed to be the man, should be able to earn enough to support the others. As a consequence, of course, single men benefited but wages and opportunities for the many women who stayed in the labour market were depressed. Some feminists argue that this led to marriage and domestic labour being the only options for many working-class women. As in the exclusion of women from 'indecent' mines, we again see women's sexuality being defined by statute or economic pressure.

In the long run, it was beneficial also to the capitalist class to have their (male) employees better fed and looked after. In other words, women came to be defined in terms of reproducing the workforce, through bearing and rearing children and caring for men. Coote and Campbell (1982) argue that the consciousness of the family wage ideology still affects trade union bargaining to the detriment of demands for equal pay.

In general, we will not look in as much detail as this at employment or wage policies but the impact of the above on women's welfare is crucial. Their assumed dependence on men was, for example, later institutionalized in the National Insurance system.

The academic response to the new Poor Law

The empirical tradition

The theory of the 1834 Act asserted that society and the economy operated naturally in the interests of all. That is, if left alone by government, trade unions, or excessive charity. Its theory was that poverty was self-inflicted or induced by the giving of relief; its solution was deterrence and the withdrawal of relief, except under extreme circumstances.

Pinker (1971) has noted that very few sociologists accepted this theory of society as valid, except Spencer who was more popular in America. Nonetheless few social theorists sought to influence government policy by challenging it or proposing alternative theories of society.

The main academic response to laissez-faire was an extremely empirical or factual one, studying the poor with a mixture of horror, anxiety, and concern. The new subject of statistics was used in many official reports, commissions of inquiry, and general recording of social phenomena in government 'blue books'. In 1857 the National Association for the Promotion of Social Science was set up, focusing its attention on the moral rather than financial condition of the poor.

Later, in the 1880s and 1890s, Charles Booth published his massive study of London poverty. He was the first writer to talk of a poverty line. Rowntree took this idea further by utilizing the new science of nutrition. He aimed to show the extent of poverty, even in relatively prosperous York. To do this, he set a deliberately low poverty definition so he would not be accused of exaggeration. Thus while he himself believed poverty to be relative, that is based on comparison with other members of society, he employed an absolute definition based merely on the requirements of 'minimum physical efficiency'. This sparse definition, widened in surveys in 1914 and 1936, was eventually incorporated into official definitions of need in Beveridge's 1942 proposals for the welfare state. Rowntree's other aim was to show that poverty was not just the product of wasteful spending as the moralists argued. To do this, he distinguished primary poverty (insufficient income) from secondary poverty (derived from wasteful or inefficient spending). Through this division he perhaps unwittingly reinforced the social construction of distinct categories of poor: the 'deserving' and the 'undeserving'.

Other researchers, often Fabian Socialists believing in the gradual social reform route to socialism, took up this tradition of factual social investigation. Eventually, this new subject of social administration became institutionalized in the London School of Economics and elsewhere.

Social theory and sociology

By this time, the distinction between social administration and its more theoretical sister subject, sociology, was clear cut and was becoming reinforced by separate university departments or courses and different syllabuses, textbooks and outlooks. The major nineteenth and early twentieth century sociologists – Marx, Weber, Durkheim – had responded to the problems of industrialism/capitalism more theoretically, seeking to analyse the main themes of social change. Even today, sociology is shy of involvement in social policy issues, possibly because of concern to appear 'neutral' and scientific and possibly because of an unwillingness to appear as a mere servicer of the practice of social administration. The significance that the social policy/problem areas of education and deviancy have for sociology makes this shyness all the more surprising.

Many writers have criticized the often narrow, administrative focus of social policy. By focusing on state services and how they deal with the poor, it has tended to ignore the question of the rich and of taxation. Field (1981) quotes Tawney as warning that 'what thoughtful rich people call the problem of poverty, thoughtful poor people call with equal justice the problem of riches'. These critics of conventional social policy studies argue that to explore welfare provision adequately, we need to look at benefits distributed through the tax system, through employment, and the welfare impact of government economic policy.

The Poor Law era

Returning now to the period and practice of the New Poor Law, we should note the following background changes in nineteenth century Britain. There were reforms in local government, public health, factory inspection, and education. Some of these were associated with attempts to appeal to those better-off sections of the male working class who achieved the vote in 1867 and 1884. Our main theme here, however, is the operation of the Poor Law itself.

Poor Law practice – continuity and change

There was much working-class hostility to the new Act and

the workhouses ('Bastilles'). As it turned out, however, there was much continuity between pre- and post-1834. Firstly, the local Poor Law guardians (mainly middle class) found that the centralized administration did not erode their power as much as they had feared. Secondly, outdoor relief continued to be given, especially in industrial areas when trade slumps made the idea of frightening the unemployed into work more than usually inappropriate.

Some historians believe that it was only in the 1860s that the Poor Law was organized on its strictly intended lines. A series of poor winters and a depression in the cotton industry led to big increases in spending on outdoor relief and charity. There was also growing concern with the condition both of children and of sick inmates of workhouses. Many commentators argued that these large institutions were breeding grounds for disease, institutional dependence, and stigma, undermining children's chances of achieving an independent life outside the workhouse. As a result, a number of changes were brought in.

Firstly, workhouse organization was tightened up. The Poor Law Board became a full department of state and, in 1871, was amalgamated with public health provision to become the Local Government Board. There were also moves to provide separate infirmaries for the sick and boarding-out arrangements for children, in theory leaving the able-bodied pauper to face the harsher workhouse test that was introduced and which lasted until the 1880s.

Secondly, concern that charity had grown indiscriminately and was demoralizing the poor gave rise to a more disciplined approach to giving. The Charity Organization Society was set up in 1869 to help regulate charity according to the Victorian virtue of self-help; charity was denied to those deemed incapable of such. The casework assessment involved in this was the forerunner of much modern social work practice and partly explains the origin of the view of social workers as agents for imposing middle-class values on the poor.

Poor Law ideals under attack

By the 1880s and 1890s, there was increasing opposition to Poor Law ideals. There was the growing organization of unskilled workers into unions, the reappearance of socialist ideas and the growth in influence of the newly enfranchized sections of the working class. Golding and Middleton (1982) note that, although class conflict and consciousness were increasing, the relatively new popular press did not express this. These papers sometimes called for reforms for 'the deserving poor' but made no criticism of overall class inequality and capitalism.

In ruling circles there was growing concern that a disaffected working class could be a threat to order and stability. Some politicians began to accept the need for reform as a ransom for the protection of privilege. In addition, whilst the new Poor Law might have been appropriate for securing the readiness to work of a large unskilled workforce new to waged labour, it was not appropriate for securing the support of an increasingly skilled workforce.

In this way welfare came to be less repressive and more ideological in its role. This distinction is based on the work of the modern French Marxist Althusser. He saw repression (by the law or armed forces) and ideological conditioning (especially through education) as ways in which the state acts to uphold the system by which most wealth is in the hands of a minority and the majority work for them. An important part of this process is getting the subordinate class to accept their position; they are more likely to do this if welfare has narrowed some of the extremes of inequality.

Concern about national efficiency

Towards the end of the century, concern was growing that Britain's main competitors, Prussia and America, were beginning to threaten her economic and imperial power. It was argued that a strong nation needed fit, healthy workers and this might require an extension of welfare provision. Behind this also was a re-working of the theory of Social Darwinism, no longer stressing the survival of the fittest individual but rather that of the group or nation; in this way Social Darwinism took on overtly racist dimensions.

It is worth noting here that Bismarck's Prussia had a more advanced education and welfare system than Britain. In introducing compulsory worker's insurance, between 1881 and 1889, Bismarck sought to win the loyalty of the German working class away from trade unionism and socialism. Its early introduction in Prussia also illustrates how the pattern of state social policy in the *period of industrialization* is affected by the dominant industrializing class. Bourgeois or entrepreneurial classes – as in America and Britain – were opposed to state interventionism. Where the dominant industrializing class was a traditional or dynastic one – as in Prussia and Japan – ideas of paternalism and protection are stronger. Interestingly, while Japan ranks low on international comparisons of state spending on welfare, its large companies often play a cradle-to-grave role in welfare provision.

British welfare development also received a boost when anxieties about national decline were heightened by evidence of massive ill health during recruitment to the Boer War (1899–1902).

Most of these explanations of welfare development in Britain roughly correspond with those of post-war Marxist historian John Saville, whose theory stressed three main factors:

(i) Property owners' recognition that welfare was necessary as a ransom for their security.

(ii) Industrial capitalism's requirement of an efficient workforce.

(iii) Working-class struggle, which has been the main determinant of the pace of reform. The other factors remind us that reforms need not be against capitalist interests.

Other explanations – progress and bureaucracy?

Some writers have argued that welfare development was a humanitarian reaction to the horrors of the Poor Law. This derives from a Whig view of history as the expression of growing enlightenment down to the present day rather than the result of conflict, struggle, and action. It also implies an uncritical view of the modern welfare state, overlooking continued poverty and inequality. More specifically, in relation to the nineteenth century itself, Fraser (1973) points to continuing complaints about the alleged softness of the Poor Law and refers to the *Daily Telegraph* in 1866 warning that any improvement to workhouse conditions could undermine the work ethic. Golding and Middleton (1982) note the 1905 *Daily Mail* story referring to the Camberwell workhouse as 'The Workhouse De Luxe', a poverty palace. Another contemporary complained that the statutory right to compensation for an accident at work (1897) reduced the worker's freedom to bargain with his employer for a rate that reflected the work's dangers.

Another set of explanations suggests that, from the 1834 Commissioners down to Beveridge, welfare state development has been the impetus of the administrators themselves, a kind of self-sustained bureaucratic initiative. This view partly stems from a methodological weakness in such approaches, namely an over-reliance on the evidence of official documents, which 'inevitably inflated the role of civil servants' (Davidson and Lowe 1981). These writers also note the sociological research that shows how bureaucracies tend to develop set routines, veer towards caution, and find innovation difficult. In the nineteenth century civil service, reliance on 'gentlemen' rather than policy specialists reinforced this. One major exception was the Labour Department which set up labour exchanges and minimum wage machinery (1909), the origin of today's wages councils in a range of low paid industries.

Alternatives to Poor Law provision – trade unions, friendly societies, and insurance companies

Outside the Poor Law system there were two main kinds of organized relief:

(i) Mutual aid. This was the collective provision in the form of contribution-based benefits made by the working class, or at least its better-off members. Mutual aid was largely organized through trade unions and friendly societies. The latter with four million members in 1872 was far more statistically significant, but less socially threatening to the powers-that-be than the trade unions.

(ii) Private insurance. The commercial insurance companies with their aggressive sales methods catered mainly for those who feared the stigma of a pauper funeral.

The twentieth century

It is often assumed that social reform is a socialist measure to be associated at party level with Labour. Indeed, the theory of Fabian Socialism directly sees reform as the route to the abolition of the capitalist system. We have already seen, however, that Marxists argue that many reforms can actually reinforce capitalism. They point to the many reforms introduced by Conservative and Liberal governments as evidence of this. The Liberal Government of 1906 was just such a reforming government.

The Liberals inherited from their Conservative predecessors a Commission of Inquiry into the Poor Laws, whose members came up with two conflicting reports in 1909, a cautious Majority Report and a more radical anti-Poor Law one, largely written by the Webbs, the most influential of the Fabians. Neither was acted upon, however, as actions by the Liberal Government made them obsolete.

Old age pensions

Firstly, after three decades of interest and agitation, Britain finally introduced old age pensions in 1908, nearly ten years after New Zealand. The pension was means tested and small and, whilst it distinguished between the 'deserving' and 'undeserving' (those who habitually failed to work or save), it was outside the hated Poor Law. Unlike today's pensions, it was financed out of general taxation with no contributory requirement. In those days, taxation extended far less into lower income groups and so pension funding had some vertical redistributive effect, that is from rich to poor.

The National Insurance Act, 1911

This introduced compulsory insurance (with contributions from employers, employees, and the state). Part I of the Act covered health insurance for all manual workers and non-manual workers below a certain income. It provided sick pay and free medical treatment from a 'panel' doctor for the worker but not his dependants. In Britain today, we take free GP or hospital treatment for granted but it is a benefit which in other times or places would have to be paid for; it is therefore called part of the social, as opposed to money, wage. Part II covered unemployment but included only 2¼ million, predominately male workers in a limited range of occupations.

Many socialists opposed the scheme because its contribution principle 'followed Bismarck's example of paying for social reform mainly out of the pockets of the poor' (Cole and Postgate 1956). It was thus a form of horizontal distribution, from the healthy and employed to the sick or unemployed.

Originally it was also opposed by friendly societies and insurance companies but they, along with trade unions, were to become 'approved societies' who would operate the system. In the long run insurance companies gained whereas the non-profit-making friendly societies were never again the force they had been (Kincaid 1975).

Generally business organizations were divided on the scheme. Some, such as the Birmingham Chamber of Commerce, followed the German example of seeing social policy as a way of responding to the strains and conflicts of industrial change. However,

'In the aftermath of the First World War, when it appeared that welfare had not yielded the productivity increases or the political peace, it was very quickly dropped as a positive strategy by those very groups of employers who had been active in support of welfare in Britain and Germany before 1914.'

(Hay 1981)

Some companies, particularly Quaker firms such as Rowntree's, already supported worker welfare schemes.

Many other companies strongly opposed National Insurance and set up an Employers' Parliamentary Association, the forerunner of the modern business pressure group the Confederation of British Industry.

Other commentators opposed the degree of bureaucratic regulation as un-British and, indeed, the amount of other 'lawlessness' at the time (Suffragettes, industrial unrest, and in Ulster) made some wonder whether the public would comply with regulations.

Finally, we need to emphasize the scheme's focus on working-class men, rather than women. Wilson (1977) notes that a scheme for a widowed mother's allowance was dropped for this reason. Fraser (1973) notes the exclusion of the worker's dependants from the provision for free medical treatment and reproduces a 1910 quote from a government official, referred to originally by Bentley Gilbert:

'Married women living with their husbands need not be included since where the unit is the family, it is the husband's and not wife's health which it is important to insure. So long as the husband is in good health and able to work, adequate provision will be made for the needs of the family, irrespective of the wife's health, whereas when the husband's health fails there is no-one to earn the wages.'

Activity

List the factual and moral assumptions about men, women, and the family made by this quote. Are they applicable today?

Further reading

The New Society Social Studies Reader The Origins of the Social Services *provides a good factual background to this period, looking at social security, housing, health, education, and factory reform.*

For a discussion of the position of women in Victorian society see Wilson (1977).

Fraser (1973) is extremely useful for those interested in a more detailed history.

For a critical account of Rowntree's approach to defining poverty and its later influence on Beveridge, see Kincaid (1975), pages 49–61.

4

Raw deal and New Deal – war, depression, and social policy

From 1914 to 1945 the Western world experienced two world wars and a major economic depression. Each had a considerable impact on the development of social policy and this is outlined below, along with various sociological theories seeking to explain this welfare development.

World War One: racism, taxation, and social policy

Wars are not usually pursued in order to change social policy but, like other social phenomena, they have many unforeseen or unintended consequences. School meals, for example, were introduced after army recruitment during the Boer War had exposed massive ill health and undernourishment in the working class: poverty had become a military problem.

Our discussion of World War One and social policy centres around three issues, chosen for their relevance to later debates.

(i) *Immigration, racism, and poverty*

One of the by-products of World War One was a growth of racism and xenophobia, especially against people with German-sounding names. This directly reinforced the anti-Semitic campaign against immigration which had, since the turn of the century, focused hostility on Jewish refugees and their poverty. Coupled with fears about national security, it led to the passing of the 1914 Aliens Registration Act, supposedly an emergency wartime measure but which was effectively re-passed every year until 1971.

Under this law an order was made in 1920 that aliens could be refused entry if they could not show the ability to support themselves and their families. They could also be deported if, within a year of arrival, they had been in receipt of poor relief or found wandering with no clear means of support. This order, which lasted until 1953, directly linked wealth with rights of movement. It also gave poor people who were aliens fewer rights than poor people who were not since the former risked deportation if they claimed poor relief. The links between racism and the social security system are discussed again on page 87 and pages 122 to 128.

It should be noted that the term 'alien' does not cover Commonwealth citizens for whom there was no statutory control until 1962.

Further reading

For a discussion of these and modern anti-immigrant campaigns and their link to the process of racist scapegoating, see Nugent and King (1979).

(ii) *Public spending and taxation*

Wars are expensive. British government spending rose tenfold from 1914 to 1916. With this came a massive increase in taxation.

Wide inequalities of wealth and income mean that certain groups have little money to tax and others a great deal. The government was also concerned that the increase in taxation should be seen to be fair so as to retain popular support for the war. It did this partly by a system of tax allowances for children. Initially, only those with incomes under £700 per year could qualify. The allowance for a wife came in 1918 and personal allowances generally in 1920. Subsequently all taxpayers could claim these allowances, regardless of their income, and in the 1950s those on high incomes were given the right to claim their allowances against their higher tax rates. Thus the rich gain more in tax relief than those on average or low incomes. This 'tax allowance Welfare State' is discussed more on pages 64 to 65.

Further reading

For a fuller account of tax allowances and their impact on the distribution of income, see Field (1981), Chapter 7.

(iii) *Hearts, minds, and social welfare*

Another important issue is the way that governments sometimes offer reforms as a means of winning the public's support for war or of expressing the increased social solidarity that war may bring. This is discussed more fully in relation to World War Two on pages 50 to 51. We should note, however, that this period saw extensions of the vote, proposals for educational reform, and 'homes fit for heroes' as well as the setting up of a Ministry of Reconstruction which, in fact, did little but was symbolic of a growing concern with matters of social policy. Economic depression, from 1920 onwards, led to many of these proposals being dropped.

Welfare for all? The spread of social insurance

Background ideas: approaches to welfare

One of the key developments of twentieth century social policy, in Britain and elsewhere, was the spread of social insurance schemes. At first, these were only for limited sections of the population, such as manual workers, but later they came to cover nearly all social groups. Insurance schemes give benefits as of right based on contributions and require no assessment of need based on income. In this way recipients are not treated as paupers or 'the poor' but remain seen as citizens who, by virtue of being sick or retired, are in receipt of an insurance benefit.

This new approach sees welfare provision, like education, as a central feature of the state's responsibility for the collective good and is therefore called the institutional approach to welfare. It is to be contrasted with the residual approach which seeks to restrict welfare provision to those who can establish their poverty. The residual approach sees the general way that market forces distribute wages, salaries, and profits as basically sound and to be interfered with as little as possible. The institutional approach sees welfare provision as a way of countering the inequality inherent in market forces. Marxism rejects both approaches and calls for major structural changes in society, including the abolition of market forces; see Chapter 6.

Both the residual and institutional approaches to welfare continued to exist side by side, though based on conflicting principles. Today in Britain, Supplementary Benefit is very much in the residual mould – giving stigmatized benefits based on established poverty – whereas old age pensions, for example, are given to all insured persons as of right.

Britain and the inter-war years: dole, depression, and the threat of revolution

From the end of 1920 until 1939, unemployment in Britain hardly fell below one million. By today's standards perhaps this figure does not appear large but the enormity of the slump can be shown by the percentage figures of British unemployment given in *Table 1*.

Table 1 *Unemployment in Britain 1921–85*

	average unemployment	maximum	minimum
	%	%	%
1921–40	14.0	22.5	10.9
1941–70	1.5	2.4	0.4
1971–80	4.0	5.8	2.3
1981–85	11.2	13.1	9.1

Source: Oxford Review of Economic Policy Vol. 1 No. 2 (OUP)

As a result, social policy came to be dominated by the question of unemployment and unemployment benefit. Other developments did occur, however, most notably the 1925 introduction of contributory pensions for widows, orphans, and the elderly. There were also a number of campaigns by women's organizations, including early demands for family allowances.

The rapid onset of high unemployment meant that the National Insurance unemployment scheme, which had been extended from its original coverage of 2¼ million workers to 11 million by 1921, ran into enormous difficulties. The National Insurance Fund had received too little in contributions to cope with the extra demand. In addition many workers were unemployed for much longer than the scheme envisaged and they ran out of entitlement to benefit.

The government feared that poverty and unemployment

would cause unrest or revolution. There was already growing conflict between employers and workers and the worry, in government circles, that the Russian Revolution of 1917 could set an example to British workers. They were keen, therefore, to provide at least some relief for the unemployed but did not want to undermine the insurance principle. Thus, they introduced uncovenanted or extended benefit, nicknamed the dole. It was supposedly a withdrawal against future contributions but was much more like a demeaning handout. It produced, says Fraser (1973), 'a demoralised nation, not a revolutionary one', though campaigns and marches against unemployment did take place – often harried by the police. E. Wilson (1977) argues that the men who were demoralized were just 'the visible part of an iceberg; sunk below them were millions of toiling, downtrodden women, their lives the picture of the most dreadful neglect'.

Further reading

For a committed social observer's view of the 1930s depression in the North of England, see Orwell (1970). For a feminist view of the 1980s depression in the same area, see Campbell (1984).

The dominant agenda from parliamentary leaderships and press alike was that taxation was a burden, especially on the middle class, and that public spending should be constantly scrutinized. It was backed up by a definition of many unemployed claimants as 'the undeserving poor'.

An example of this scrutiny came in 1927 with the extension of entitlement to benefit to those of the long term unemployed whose qualification for benefit had run out. In order to qualify they had to prove that they were genuinely seeking work. This test was clearly derived from a definition of unemployment as the product of individual psychology rather than economic circumstances. Given the massive collapse of industries it was simply a further blow to the self-esteem of the unemployed worker.

Though this system was modified in 1930, the world-wide financial collapse of 1931 led to increased unemployment and a further harsh response from government. This time, benefit rates were cut and the rigorous household means test was introduced, looking into the needs, income, and circumstances of all the household members of an applicant for dole. It took account of any money that retired household members had and adjusted the dole accordingly; it was seen as intrusive and became the cause of many family conflicts. 'Like the work-house before it, it was destined to leave an indelible mark on popular culture' (Fraser 1973).

During all this time, the Poor Law continued to function as a last resort relief agency, though some Poor Law Guardians, notably in Poplar, were considered too generous. As a result, the government reduced their powers (1926) and then transferred them to local authority Public Assistance Committees (1929). When the Unemployment Assistance Board was set up in 1934 and benefit levels restored, the Poor Law effectively lost all concern for the able-bodied poor.

There were also, in the 1930s, some public works schemes designed to stimulate employment but they were not very effective. Their main advocate, the economist J. M. Keynes, left England for America where he had a significant influence on the social and economic initiative called the New Deal.

Sociological note: C. Wright Mills, private troubles, and public issues

Whilst Mills was an American sociologist of the post World War Two period, his writings on what he called the sociological imagination can be applied directly to an understanding of the 'genuinely seeking work' test or anywhere that social problems, such as poverty or unemployment, are explained in individual or psychological terms. It was his view that the application of the sociological imagination to the understanding of social problems can be considerably aided by distinguishing between 'personal troubles of milieu' and 'public issues of social structure'.

Personal troubles concern an individual's biography and immediate personal relationships; public issues are wider matters of history and society, its values, class system, and institutions. Mills (1970) contrasts a city of 100,000 people where one person in unemployed as an example of a personal trouble to be explained perhaps in terms of that person's character with a nation of 50 million workers where 15 million of them are unemployed, which is a public issue:

> 'we may not hope to find its solution within the range of opportunities open to any one individual. The very structure of opportunities has collapsed. Both the correct statement of the problem and the range of possible solutions require us to consider the economic and political institutions of the society, and not merely the personal situation and character of a scatter of individuals.'

To define public issues constantly as personal problems is effectively to blame individuals for circumstances outside their influence and can, therefore, be seen as an ideology of social control.

American society and social welfare

Depression and New Deal – the background

Early twentieth century America had seen some calls for social insurance, especially for workmen's compensation for industrial injury. Its main supporters were civic leaders, professionals in the social work field, and those managements which saw labour as an economic resource to be valued, preserved, and strengthened; for them economic rationality involved support for some progressive social policies. Opposition to such schemes was considerable, however, for social insurance was seen to clash with the dominant American ideology of individualism and self-reliance.

In particular social insurance was opposed because it smacked of German authoritarian paternalism, especially after World War One had increased anti-German sentiment. It was also opposed by those who associated it with what they saw as British egalitarianism; many companies, in particular, saw social insurance as a step towards socialism, something they vehemently opposed. Insurance companies saw it as a threat to their own private business. Trade unions viewed it as a diversion from the 'real' struggle over wages and conditions, seeing their organizations and workers as too rugged and self-reliant to need social insurance. Mishra (1981) notes, however, that these unions in The American Federation of Labor were largely white, male, and skilled and therefore less likely to suffer low wages or unemployment – at least until the 1930s. The absence of unions for the unskilled workers until the Congress of Industrial Organization in the 1930s is, he says, a more significant factor in the 'welfare laggard' status of the US than the ideology of individualism itself.

The social insurance campaign died down in the prosperous 1920s, a decade of supposed 'welfare capitalism' where people's needs were increasingly to be met through their conditions of employment. In fact, however, by 1930 only 10 per cent of America's over sixty-fives were on a pension, of which about 80 per cent were military pensions. Under ½ per cent were in unemployment schemes. The only other provision was workmen's compensation and the stigmatized almshouse, catering for about 100,000 people in 1930.

Thus America was ill-prepared for the depression which, arriving later than Britain's, came in 1929 after financial collapse on America's stock exchange. However, the depression rapidly became more severe than Britain's ever was: from 1929 to 1933 output fell by one-third and unemployment reached 15 million (29 per cent of the workforce); it also had a devastating effect on farm prices and incomes.

Further reading

John Steinbeck's The Grapes of Wrath *(1951) provides a powerful, fictional account of the collapse of opportunity and the repression of the poor set against acute agricultural poverty. The film is also worth seeing.*

The depression also brought a decline in charitable poor relief and reduced the ability of the worst hit areas to provide their own schemes. People's faith in laissez-faire was challenged. Earlier theorists had seen economic slumps as invigorating, killing off weak and inefficient companies; see the section on Spencer and Sumner on page 20. Increasingly, however, some kind of state action came to be seen as necessary but it took until Roosevelt's 1935 New Deal for it to arrive.

Despite the pressure for reform there remained considerable hostility to state intervention in general and the New Deal in particular. Baran and Sweezey refer to opposition from 'the power structure of monopoly capitalism'. Gouldner (1971) places middle-class hostility to the New Deal in terms of a wider crisis causing acute anxiety within the American and international middle class:

(i) World War One had shattered bourgeois confidence and its belief in automatic progress.

(ii) The rise of fascism in Europe and communism in Russia led to fears of unrest and revolution.

(iii) The depression itself brought a crisis of confidence in America's values and institutions.

(iv) Finally, to many in the middle class, the proposed New Deal reforms in social welfare, industrial relations, employment practices, and economic policy were worse than the depression itself. They feared the New Deal more than Marxism for the latter was attractive only to a minority. Many spoke with hatred of Roosevelt 'even though the point of the New Deal reforms was to stabilise the established system in its essentials rather than overturn it' (Gouldner 1971).

The New Deal arrives

The main components of Roosevelt's 1935 welfare legislation were: aid for the elderly, unemployment insurance, public assistance, and aid for the blind.

The case of the elderly is interesting partly because, unlike in Europe, pension provision did not precede their significant growth as a proportion of the overall population. This meant that, along with the jolt from the depression and its attendant hardships, this provision was pushed along by the size of the elderly electorate. Rimlinger (1971) notes, however, that 'the high cost of relief in poor houses became, perhaps, the most powerful force favouring old age pensions'.

The provision itself was based on two schemes: a slow-to-mature insurance scheme which Roosevelt sought to 'sell' to the opposition on the basis of its American values of helping oneself and looking to the future; secondly, a means-tested system which was sold on its strictness and which was finally abolished in 1971 by which time few relied on it. Interestingly, a third proposal, a voluntary scheme for a higher level of pension, was dropped because of opposition from private insurance companies. A final point of interest is that southern states pressed for a low basic level of provision for the elderly so that elderly blacks did not get more than the whites felt justifiable.

Unemployment insurance was always more opposed than pension insurance. The depression and the change in their membership brought American trade unions round to supporting it but the Republican Party remained opposed and business continued to be very sceptical. For a while, the constitutional division of powers between federal and state government held up nationally imposed schemes but the 1935 Act overcame this and, by 1937, every state had an unemployment insurance scheme though state autonomy did undermine the scheme's effectiveness. Rimlinger says such constitutional opposition to federal control was often 'a screen for the resistance of the business community to the extension of social rights'. This is a classic example of ideology at work: defending a vested interest but claiming to be acting in line with some higher principle or the interests of all society.

Many of the justifications of the New Deal were framed in the language of American ideals. Thus unemployment insurance was defined as a protection of individualism and family life under threat from the long term absence of work. Equally, mass poverty was seen as bad for the economy since it undermined consumer demand for goods; this can be seen as the influence of Keynes's theories. In many ways, the values of the market place were more significant than need or justice, both in the shaping of policy and in its legitimating ideologies. For example, the lack of coverage in the scheme for widows, orphans, and workers' families 'can be traced to the values of a society that idealized the cash nexus' (Rimlinger 1971). Furthermore when, in 1939, social security was extended to family protection this was not seen to clash with the ideology of individualism since this belief assumed men would be competitive individuals and women would be dependants located in the family. For a discussion of this 'family wage' issue, see pages 21 to 22.

There were other major gaps in the New Deal, notably family allowances and a national system of health insurance, the latter omission largely indicating the powerful conservative influence of the American Medical Association. Nonetheless the New Deal remains the most important step in social reform ever undertaken by an American government, as is perhaps indicated by the continued absence of either family allowances or a national health insurance scheme. Interestingly Canada introduced the former in 1944 and the latter in 1971, confirming its slightly less laggard status than America; see page 19 for an earlier explanation of this.

Welfare explanations: the case of America

Conflict perspectives

Conflict perspectives in sociology argue that different groups in society have different economic and other interests, often leading to differences of outlook and ideology. Social policy is analysed in terms of which groups' interests it serves. Here we look at conflict perspectives on American welfare developments; later, in Chapter 6, we explore more fully two major examples of the conflict perspective: feminism and Marxism.

We have already seen, on page 27, how the Marxist perspective on welfare stresses both the way in which reforms can be used to strengthen capitalism and yet many only come about after working-class struggle against capitalist opposition. Some writers emphasize both equally, but others stress the importance of one factor over the other. The American radicals Piven and Cloward actually move from stressing the first, the way reforms reinforce capitalist interests, to the second, how they express working-class pressure.

In a 1972 book, they argued that American welfare had, over the years, tended to expand when disorder threatened but, when employers needed a ready supply of cheap labour, it contracted to make low paid work more palatable. In a 1982 book, they stressed the degree to which welfare is more in the interests of the working class and expands with struggles to make the economy more accountable to the needs of the people. Underlying this latter argument is the view that the capitalist market rewards those with capital or strong labour-market positions but those without either lose out. These tend to be the unskilled or poorly unionized sections of the workforce, or black and women workers.

In their 1982 approach they claim that, until the depression, the dominance of laissez-faire ideology prevented any significant growth in American welfare. The New Deal is seen as a kind of victory of democratic political pressure over capitalism which led to the entrenchment of the idea of government responsibility for welfare provision and the workings of the economy – something which President Reagan is aiming to reverse.

Functionalist perspectives

The functionalist perspective in sociology is based on certain assumptions about the nature of society. Firstly, society is seen as composed of a number of inter-related parts, each playing a part (its function) in maintaining the overall system or structure. This view, even if over-simplified here, has led many functionalists to argue against deliberate social change since the inter-relatedness of the system will mean that changes in one area will have unforeseen and possibly disastrous consequences somewhere else. Thus many functionalists tend towards political conservatism and, indeed, Talcott Parsons, the leading mid-twentieth century American functionalist, was strongly opposed to the New Deal reforms.

A second major assumption of functionalism is that society is based on a commitment to shared values. In general they stress order, cohesion and consensus. Thus when America's traditional values seemed threatened by depression, rather than seek a solution through social and economic reform, like the New Deal, Parsons called for a strengthening of individual commitment to the cherished values of individualism and self-reliance.

In general, however, functionalism is neither necessarily pro- nor anti-welfare. We have already seen how the nineteenth century functionalist and Social Darwinist Herbert Spencer opposed welfare reforms as interfering with the assumed evolutionary advance of society towards higher forms. Many other functionalists, however, have stressed the role of reform in the promotion of social integration. They often see welfare as a societal adaptation to the stresses of industrialism; functionalists tend to assume that societies have a natural tendency to seek equilibrium.

Durkheim, for example, saw social welfare as a means of

promoting social solidarity, which had been weakened by industrialization, urbanization, and the growth of competitive individualism. These forces had led to a decline of moral discipline on individuals and an increasing tendency for them to have unrealistic expectations of life – a condition that he called anomie. For Durkheim this was a bigger problem than poverty; in fact, he saw the rigours and disciplines of poverty as somewhat of a solution to anomie.

The question of social solidarity is a central theme in a later section – the debate over the influence of World War Two on British social policy.

World War Two – history, sociology, and the individual

The discussion of British social policy during and after World War Two raises two general questions of the sociological perspective: the relationship between history and sociology; the importance that sociologists attach to individual action rather than social forces or groups.

History and sociology

The issues raised here are not just relevant to this period or chapter but indicate the importance of history to sociology and, it is hoped, will show that the early chapters of this book are more than just historical background. They are important not only in understanding how social policy came to be as it is today but also the general nature of welfare itself.

The first issue is that of causes. The search for explanations in sociology leads us to look at what preceded an event or social development. Social policy in particular is often a conscious response to a previous social development, like disorder or the threat of it. We also have to look at the unintended consequences of social action, as we did in the discussion of World War One, and shall do about World War Two.

Secondly, and related to the first, is the question of

comparison. Unless we compare societies, either from different places or periods, we cannot discover the circumstances usually associated with the phenomenon in question, and those which are not. Without this, generalization is much more difficult. Generalization involves not just asking what happened to British social policy at the time of World War Two but seeking to find the connections between these two events. It also means asking about general links between war and social policy and, further still, what this tells us about the general nature of the role of welfare in society.

Sociology and the individual – social policy and charisma?

So far our explanations of welfare development have largely been in terms of broad social forces, such as class conflict or the influence of belief systems. This is to be expected in a sociology text. Occasional reference has been made, however, to the contribution of individuals, such as Malthus. Social reform after World War Two is enormously associated with the name of Beveridge, writer of the government report *Social Insurance and Allied Services* (1942), which has sold 750,000 copies – a staggering number for an official document.

What does this suggest about the influence of individuals on social change? How does it affect our view that social policy developments are largely to do with structural or ideological forces, rather than a 'great' man or woman? At a general level, the historian E. H. Carr has argued that such an individual 'is always representative either of existing forces or of forces which he helps to create by way of challenge to existing authority' (Carr 1964). Usually it is the social forces rather than the individual which interest the sociologist.

The idea of such individuals was recognized, however, by the sociologist Max Weber. In his analysis of political authority he outlined three ways in which those in positions of power gain acceptance or legitimacy for their dominance. One is based on tradition, as in the case of hereditary monarchs. Another is the authority that comes from holding a position or office which is governed by rules and regulations that are generally considered legitimate. This rational-legal authority is associated with the spread of bureaucracy, often the very type of organization associated with the growth of welfare provision. Thirdly, Weber used the term 'charisma' to describe the position where a person gains authority from the personal qualities he or she is seen to have. Interesting here, in view of Carr's comment above, is the fact that charisma does not derive solely from the individual but rather it is a product of large numbers of people believing a person to have certain qualities. In that way, the leader is representative of social forces as well as part creator of them and, in the language of sociology, charisma can be seen to be socially constructed.

In terms of Weber's analytic framework, charisma facilitates innovation whereas bureaucracy makes it more difficult. He was aware, however, and many studies have shown, that bureaucracies are seldom as formal and impersonal as the abstract model would suggest. Individuals can and do make their mark, and not just 'great' ones. At the level of policy making, one historical study of bureaucracy and innovation in British social policy has suggested that the growth in size and the standardization of its recruitment has reduced the potential for innovation in the civil service. It also points to a methodological problem in making such observations; namely that the tradition of civil service anonymity has inhibited research into that area. The authors, Davidson and Lowe (1981), conclude that innovation in British civil service history has depended on an exceptional individual. Clearly, many see Beveridge as such a person though Kincaid argues that it is not as a visionary that Beveridge deserves to be remembered. 'Rather his particular distinction lay in an ability to translate the general objectives of ruling-class reformism into detailed and technically workable proposals' (Kincaid 1975).

War, reform, and social solidarity

Richard Titmuss has been one of the main exponents of the view that World War Two brought a major shift in British social policy. He places this in a general overview of the relationship between war and state concern for the condition of the people (Titmuss 1958). This concern starts with biological factors: numbers of men available for battle and their fitness, leading on to questions of the breeding and rearing of the next generation of potential soldiers. He notes that in the nineteenth century there was much opposition to census operations because of possible military motives.

This concern moves on to questions of the social condition of soldiers and civilians, at least where the war has a major impact on them as the 'total' wars of 1914–18 and 1939–45 clearly did. Reforms, or the promise of them, often play a part in retaining civilian support for war. This leads into Andreski's (1964) theory of the link between war and social inequality. On the basis of research from pre-literate and advanced industrial societies, Andreski argues that, where the mass of the population are involved in a war, social inequalities tend to decrease. However, where wars are fought by professional soldiers, recruited from a social elite, the war tends to widen inequalities. In the latter case, it seems, the rulers do not have to win the support of the populace.

In terms of World War Two, Titmuss argues that it influenced social policy in three ways:

(i) Popular opinion was affected by the shared vulnerability of war and social solidarity was enhanced by opposition to a common enemy. This reduced many people's opposition to egalitarian and collectivist policies.

(ii) As middle-class families in country areas took in poor and working-class children evacuated from the bombed cities, there was a spread of information about the degree of poverty and general nature of social problems.

(iii) The government was willing to respond to these because it wanted a fit, nourished, efficient, and contented nation. This response is represented by the Beveridge Report.

Further reading

For elaboration of these ideas on war and social policy see Titmuss (1958) and, for a different point of view, Harris (1981).

The Beveridge Report

The Beveridge Report grew out of a committee on social insurance, especially workmen's compensation, that Beveridge was put in charge of in 1941. It became a major critique of the five giant evils of Squalor, Disease, Ignorance, Idleness, and Want, as well as a plan for their solution.

Rather than receiving this with pleasure as a way of promoting social solidarity, Harris's research indicates many ministers and civil servants were alarmed about the proposals and their cost. Indeed they unsuccessfully tried to keep the committee's work quiet.

The Report was published in 1942 and, some changes and cuts aside, laid the basis of the social reforms of the post-war Labour Government and the foundations of the welfare system for the next four decades. Its key elements can be summarized as follows:

Principles and organization   The main attack on want was to be by extending National Insurance to cover (nearly) all the employed population; this was passed in 1946. The main risks covered were the established ones of old age, sickness, industrial injury, and unemployment. Benefits were to be universal and as-of-right. Contributions and benefits were to be flat rate, subsistence-level and to last as long as the need. Neither of the last two proposals was fully implemented;

benefit levels were below subsistence and benefits for the unemployed lasted only twelve months.

This meant that many people had to rely on National Assistance (renamed Supplementary Benefit in 1966) which was introduced in 1948, finally ending the Poor Law. It was means tested, subsistence based, financed out of taxation and available to those 'without resources to meet their requirements', unless they were in full-time work. In theory it was to be a safety net for a few.

For a theoretical discussion of these two types of welfare provision, see page 36.

Assumptions Beveridge argued that this attack on poverty would only work if three other policies were implemented:

(i) Government responsibility for maintaining full employment, including state spending to promote jobs (for example, council house building), even if this meant borrowing the money. This economic policy, based on the theories of Keynes, was to remain the dominant one until the 1970s.

(ii) A National Health Service to ensure good, free treatmet for all; introduced in 1948.

(iii) An allowance for children; introduced in 1945 for second and subsequent children.

Titmuss's theory would suggest that these family allowances can be understood in terms of government concern with a healthy reproduction of the population and an attack on poverty as a means of promoting efficiency and civilian morale. Research by Macnicol (1980) suggests that, whatever official ideology at the time was, the introduction of family allowances can be seen in quite different ways, such as a desire to make higher taxes and lower wage increases more acceptable.

Omissions Two groups can be specifically highlighted as being overlooked by the Beveridge proposals: women, the disabled.

Married women in employment could opt out of paying all

but a small part of their 'stamp', covering industrial injury at work. This is Beveridge's comment:

> 'During marriage most women will not be gainfully employed. The small minority of women who undertake paid employment or other gainful occupations after marriage require special treatment differing from that of a single woman. Since such paid work will in many cases be intermittent, it should be open to any married woman to undertake it as an exempt person, paying no contributions of her own and acquiring no claim to benefit in unemployment or sickness. If she prefers to contribute and to requalify for unemployment and disability benefit she may do so but will receive benefits at a reduced rate.'

Activity

What assumptions does this quote contain about:
– the role of men and women in society?
– the way income is distributed in the family?
– the degree to which welfare is concerned with meeting need?

You may find it useful here to read the sections on the 'family wage', pages 21 to 22, and feminism.

Another assumption of Beveridge's was that the divorce rate would remain stable and low. Thus there was no provision for unsupported or single mothers who therefore had to rely on National Assistance. Housewives had no right to benefit either, unless widowed and then they were to have a pension for life or until remarriage.

Secondly, there is the question of the disabled. Here the treatment of different categories of disabled people illustates clearly the way that welfare policy is concerned with values other than need. Thus the non-industrially disabled were not covered by the insurance scheme and were disadvantaged compared to those disabled at work. Two of the justifications given by Beveridge for this preferential treatment are the need to reassure workers in dangerous jobs and, secondly, the fact the the worker is acting under orders. Thus the needs of employment practice and the hierarchical nature of the workplace are determinants of benefit rather than the circumstances of the individual. Beveridge's commitment to the insurance principle meant that the congenitally disabled were overlooked since they would not be able to pay stamps.

War, reform, and consensus – the reaction to Beveridge

Beveridge's biographer, José Harris, argues (1981) that civil servants and politicians generally did not, as Titmuss argued, see welfare as a wartime morale booster; initially, at least, it was seen as 'an inconvenient luxury'.

The response from pressure groups, including those from business and the trade unions, from the mass media and from public opinion, was almost universally supportive. One exception came from those women's organizations concerned about the implications of Beveridge for women (see above). No business organization or right-wing newspaper attacked the proposals in terms of laissez-faire individualism; few trade unions or representatives of the left attacked the degree of state control involved or the fact that flat-rate contributions take proportionately more from the poor than the rich (that is, they are regressive). There did, at this level, appear to be the genuine national consensus envisaged by Titmuss (1958) as the war acted on public opinion and social solidarity. Thus welfare reform could sail ahead with little significant opposition. After the war, however, ideological diversity re-emerged and, with it, opposition to some of the principles and practices of welfare. In particular, right-wing definitions of welfare as a tax/public burden were to resurface, though until recently there was no major attempt to dismantle the welfare provision made in the wake of Beveridge.

The Beveridge welfare package and commitment to full employment were part of what has been called 'the post-war settlement' between the classes, after the intense division and conflict of the inter-war years. The challenge to and breaking of this settlement is the basis of many later sections of the book.

Conclusion – Britain, welfare, and the world

Britain experienced a more rapid growth in welfare provision after World War Two than other countries at that time. By 1950, twelve times as much per head of population was being spent on social security benefits as in 1900 (Saville, 1957/8, though he argues caution in interpreting this fact). With this came the widespread acceptance of a number of questionable assumptions and responses:

(i) There was a thing called a welfare state which Britain now had and others did not.

(ii) This reinforced the academic narrowness, or even ethnocentrism, of the discipline of social administration, focusing on British welfare to the exclusion of comparison and cross-national studies.

(iii) It led to a politically complacent view that all had been achieved. Some believed a social revolution had occurred, that Britain was no longer capitalist or was even in transition to socialism. These are some of the topics that will be explored in the next chapter.

Further reading

Field (1981) and Wilson (1977) give good accounts of welfare in this and other periods of the twentieth century. The first goes into quite a lot of detail on the policies themselves; the second relates the issues to wider debates, especially the position of women in society.

5

The post-war world: growth and affluence – for some

By 1950, then, Britain had a dramatically overhauled system of state welfare. From then on the economic boom that most Western capitalist nations experienced from the 1950s to the 1970s enabled general welfare spending to increase quite rapidly despite the fact that the wartime consensus on such matters had already begun to disappear.

America, however, had no equivalent welfare expansion in the post-war period, though there were improvements in income support for the elderly. From 1949 to 1955 the percentage of the population covered by old age insurance grew from 65 per cent to 90 per cent. Heclo (1981) suggests this lack of American reform stems from a number of factors. Firstly, America had no wartime coalition or consensus on welfare. Secondly, the overlap between the questions of provision for the poor and civil rights for the black population led many racialists who opposed the latter to oppose the former as well. Thirdly, there was in America, during this cold war period, a greater stress on matters of foreign policy and national security. From this came a condemnation of anything, like welfare provision, smacking of un-Americanism and, especially, that most stigmatized of belief systems: communism.

Economic growth: gainers and losers

When looking at the consequences of this economic boom in more detail, we should bear in mind that economic growth does not benefit everyone equally. Indeed, there are costs as well as benefits to economic growth, as new industries replace old ones, bringing unemployment to certain industries or regions.

The case of Northern Ireland

The situation of Northern Ireland is a particularly interesting case in this respect. Not only did the UK have a much slower growth rate than many other countries but within the UK certain regions, especially the South-east, gained considerably and others, notably Northern Ireland, had sustained and significant levels of social and economic deprivation. John Ditch (1983) has argued that the levels of unemployment, deprivation, and conflict that today have led many to talk of a welfare crisis in Britain existed thirty years ago in Northern Ireland. Evason (1980) has recently shown that poverty is still much greater there than on most of the mainland.

In looking at the post-war situation in Northern Ireland, Ditch refers to the lack of a welfare consensus based on shared war experiences. Northern Ireland had much less involvement in the war; it had no bombing or conscription, for example. Another factor at work was the divided nature of Ireland. The partition into North and South had occurred only thirty years previously and Northern Ireland was divided on religious lines between a Protestant majority and a Roman

Catholic minority. The political role of welfare is illustrated here with the attempt, by the Protestant Unionist Party, to use reform as a way of keeping its support among working-class Protestants and even winning over some Catholics. As it turned out, however, there was strong Protestant opposition to these reforms; many Unionists (then directly linked to the Conservative Party) opposed them as too socialistic whilst there were also allegations that they were being abused by Catholics. The absence of a mass political party of the left, like the British Labour Party, which could unite the working class in demands for reform and lower levels of unemployment is a major factor in the continued deprivation in Northern Ireland.

Private wealth and public squalor

The distribution of the rewards of economic growth is not just a question of winners and losers but concerns also the distribution of the national cake between personal consumption (such as cars, holidays, clothes) and public services (health, housing, and so on). Whilst spending on the latter did increase in the 1950s, it did not do so sufficiently fast to prevent the American economist Galbraith (1970) pointing to the development of private affluence and public squalor. Our concern in this book is primarily with questions of poverty and income rather than health or housing though the two clearly interlink. Mack and Lansley (1985) note that 'Public squalor diminishes the lives of everyone in the community, poverty affects the individual and stems from that individual's lack of resources.'

Assumptions about the 1950s: all things bright and beautiful

The social comment of the 1950s often ignored the problems and inequalities associated with growth. Academics, politicians, and the mass media generally agreed that society was not only becoming better off but was also undergoing a radical change. In America, an official of Eisenhower's 1951 administration claimed that 'the transformation of the distribution of our national income . . . may already be counted as one of the great social revolutions in history'. In Britain, Anthony Crosland, Labour MP and influential social theorist, claimed in 1956 that capitalism had been 'reformed almost out of recognition'.

Marxists not only rejected the factual accuracy of these claims but saw them as ideologies masking the massive inequalities of income, wealth, and power still existing in both those capitalist societies.

The extent to which the post-war world was dominated by falsely optimistic assumptions is indicated by Townsend's (1976) observation that poverty almost disappeared from popular or academic discussion until the mid 1950s in Britain and the late 1950s in America. In so far as poverty was seen at all, it was no longer seen as a class-related experience but was increasingly referred to in terms of what are apparently quite distinct groups: the elderly, unemployed, sick, and so on. To Marxists this again was a diversion for they argued that it was not, for example, old age itself that caused poverty. Rather it was a reflection of a person's occupation before retirement and their absence of capital; in other words, class.

Marshall (1969) has noted that, as the poor came to be seen as a much smaller, even exceptional or residual group, some began to argue that the universal provision of the Beveridge scheme was no longer necessary. This view was reinforced by the imagery of malnutrition and poverty of the 1930s, leading to the assertion that post-war Britain had no 'real' poverty. This assertion, however, fails to take into account the possibility (and reality) that, while the absolute condition of the poor can and did improve, their position relative to the rest of the population could and did deteriorate.

The rest of this chapter will now explore in more detail the main arguments that changes in post-war capitalist societies, and especially the welfare state in Britain, had dramatically reduced the degree of social and economic inequality.

Activity

Watch as many British-made films from the 1940s and 1950s on television as you can bear! Watch, in particular, for themes of interclass social mixing, broken barriers, reduced inequality, and so on. Keep these images in mind when reading the rest of this chapter. How accurate do you think these images are?

The decline of inequality?

Problems of definition and measurement

There are two main issues here. What are we trying to measure? How accurate is the information available? In a pioneering work in 1958 Titmuss demonstrated the many devices that the rich use to disguise their true wealth, for tax purposes for example. It is possible then that figures on inequality of income and wealth will actually underestimate the degree of inequality.

Equally importantly, we must be clear about what it is that we are measuring. It is useful to make the following distinctions when looking at the impact of government policies on the distribution of income:

(i) Primary distribution based on market rewards: wages, salaries, profits.

(ii) Primary redistribution which takes into account direct taxes on income, gifts, inheritance, or capital gains, as well as transfer payments, primarily social security benefits.

(iii) Monetary redistribution which measures the effect of indirect taxes on people's incomes; these include VAT, customs duties, and rates.

(iv) Total redistribution includes an assessment of the differential impact of the state provision of such services as health, education, and so on. It does not mean society is totally equal.

The focus of this volume is on primary and monetary redistribution, that is the impact of taxes and cash benefits.

Activity

To illustrate the idea of total redistribution, write down which social groups you think get most benefit from (a) state education, (b) state health care. Give reasons for your answers.

You might check your ideas for (a) from any basic sociology text dealing with educational opportunity and achievement, and for (b) with Trowler (1984), pages 183–4

Trends in inequality

(i) *Income and wealth* Despite the problems of measurement, some definite trends in the distribution of income and wealth can be isolated. Kraus (1981) has argued that in Western Europe and the US from 1935 to 1950 the bottom 60 per cent increased their share of national income at the expense of the top 10 per cent. From then onwards income distribution stabilized though the top group may have improved their share slightly; this latter trend has become far more pronounced in Britain in recent years – see page 102. It is also the case that Britain's distribution of income has traditionally been far greater than comparable nations, a pattern that has probably changed little.

The failure of income distribution to become more equal or even less so after 1950 can be partly explained by changes in the labour markets of advanced capitalist societies. Bosanquet (1983) argues that reduced demand for semi- and unskilled work is significantly weakening the labour market position of those unqualified for or excluded from more skilled employment. The labour market is becoming polarized into primary workers with security, fringe benefits, possibilities of training, and so on and secondary workers with low pay, little security, few fringe benefits or chances of acquiring a skill, and high risks of unemployment. It is women and black people who are far more likely to be found in the secondary labour market; the young inner city dweller has also lost out considerably in these changes.

Similar trends were to be found in the US. Earnings of black men compared to white men slightly worsened from 1949 to 1959 while black unemployment went from being 20 per cent higher than white in 1940 and 53 per cent higher in 1953 to 112 per cent higher in 1963 (Marris and Rein 1974).

In terms of wealth distribution, looking over a longer period Atkinson and Harrison (1978) note that the top 1 per cent saw their share of personal wealth fall by half from 1923 to 1972. However, nearly all this redistribution was to the next 9 per cent; that is a transfer from the extremely rich to the very rich. By 1975 the Royal Commission on the Distribution of Income and Wealth, using a range of measurement techniques, estimated that:
- the top 1 per cent owned between 14 per cent and 24 per cent of personal wealth;
- the top 10 per cent owned between 40 per cent and 60 per cent of personal wealth;
- three-quarters of the wealth of the top 1 per cent was inherited.

Further reading

For more detail of these matters, see Field (1981) Chapters 2 and 9.

(ii) *Taxes and benefits* The post-World War Two reforms made a massive improvement in the lives of the disadvantaged. This is accepted by most Marxists who are generally sceptical of the value of reforms without abolishing capitalism.

However, they and others have pointed to the failure to abolish poverty or to redistribute from rich to poor.

They point out that social security provision, largely based on National Insurance and Supplementary Benefit, is not progressively financed. Progressive taxes are those which take proportionately more from those on higher incomes; regressive taxes are the reverse. National Insurance benefits are based on contributions. Originally they were flat-rate contributions; clearly £1 per week or whatever is worth proportionately more to a worker on £50 than one on £250. Now NI contributions are based on a percentage of earnings, though there is a 'ceiling' or earnings level above which NI contributions stop being increased.

Even that share of social security funding which comes out of taxation is not necessarily progressive. Firstly, we should distinguish between company taxation and taxation on individuals; the share of government revenue coming from the former fell from 18.4 per cent in 1946 to 7.4 per cent in 1979 bringing a shift in taxation on to individuals. This was reflected in the lowering of tax thresholds, the amount a person can earn before paying tax, to below the poverty line; thus far more working-class people became income tax payers. We need also to distinguish direct and indirect taxation; VAT is the main example of the latter and, like most taxes on commodities, takes a higher percentage of the incomes of the poor. Indirect taxes make up about 30 per cent of government revenue.

In short, much welfare provision is paid for out of the pockets of the working class themselves and the idea of the welfare state as an institutionalized Robin Hood is very misleading.

Other systems of welfare; other forms of inequality

So far discussion has concentated on the iceberg phenomenon of welfare and not looked at the less publicly recognized systems of welfare: occupational or company welfare; fiscal or tax-allowance welfare.

Occupational welfare, including such benefits as company pension schemes, sick pay, subsidized meals, cheap loans, and company cars, can be said to embrace the area known as fringe benefits or perks. These benefits grew rapidly in the post-war period. Field (1981) notes that 2.6 million workers were in occupational pension schemes in 1936, 6.2 million in 1953, 8 million in 1956 and 11.1 million in 1963. Mostly these benefits tended to reinforce conventional hierarchies based on class, income, and gender. A 1984 report by the Low Pay Unit (*Unequal Fringes*) shows that, to a company director on a basic salary of £25,000 per annum, fringe benefits can be worth an extra £12,500. *The Guardian*, 17 January, 1985, refers to a report by the London Amenity and Transport Association which estimated that tax perks for company cars cost each household in Britain about £75 per year.

Tax allowances as a form of welfare only go to those who pay direct taxes, in particular income tax. We have already seen that many low paid workers are in this category but many other poor are not; they therefore lose out on these benefits. They are benefits since money otherwise paid in tax is kept by the taxpayer. Reference has already been made to personal tax allowances for taxpayers and their dependants. Other tax allowances or concessions include the following benefits going to home owners/buyers: the abolition in 1963 of a tax on land and buildings called Schedule A tax; exemption from capital gains tax on profit from the sale of one's house; income tax relief on money paid in mortgage interest payments, even for the very rich, high-tax-rate payers. All this would be raising about £5 billion per year now and the very well off gain disproportionately from this subsidy to property owners. Until 1983, life insurance premiums attracted tax relief, though a scheme had been introduced to give reduced premiums for non-taxpayers who otherwise would have lost the benefit. Much of the provision in the occupational welfare state, especially pension schemes, attracts tax relief and these schemes are used by the highly paid to defer income to a later date when they will be paying income tax at a lower rate.

All this indicates that the estimated £20 billion lost in government revenue through tax allowances/benefits tends to favour the well paid, though research on this is incomplete. In Canada, however, the National Council of Welfare in 1976 published a detailed analysis of the situation there. It showed that the seventeen most important tax benefits cost $6.4 billion or nineteen times the cost of social security provision for the poor. This tax gain to the population gave an average of $244 to people with incomes of less than $5,000 per annum and $2,427 to those with incomes of $25,000–50,000 per annum.

The wider context – the decline of class?

Not only was it generally assumed in establishment circles that poverty was increasingly a thing of the past but it was also believed that the whole class structure was in the process of decomposition. Many writers – Zweig (1961), Abrams and Rose (1960), Crosland (1956) – became associated with the view that the incomes, living standards and lifestyles of the manual working class were becoming increasingly middle class. This was called the embourgeoisement thesis.

Clearly, in absolute terms the working class were getting better off but this does not mean that they had become or sought to become middle class. Generally the thesis implicitly assumed a superiority of middle-class culture which the working class was 'catching up' to or 'copying', which is similar to those views of the poor which assume that low income equals inferior culture and character. The main sociological opponents of this thesis, Goldthorpe and Lockwood (1969), carried out research indicating the continuation of distinctive working-class cultural patterns. Possibly more important from our point of view was the authors' stress on the need to see workers as producers as well as consumers.

65

Here they note that 'the work situation of white collar employees is still generally superior to that of manual wage earners in terms of working conditions and amenities, continuity of employment, fringe benefits, long term income prospects and promotion chances'. Thus, while there are other reasons for rejecting the embourgeoisement thesis, the inequality in company or occupational welfare provision is certainly one such reason.

It should also be noted that the similarity of earnings (consumer power) between manual and non-manual workers was often overestimated in the embourgeoisement thesis. Manual workers' wages rely more on piece work, overtime, and relative youthfulness (twenties/thirties) and they are more affected by sickness, injury, and unemployment. Comparison of weekly, as opposed to annual or lifetime, earnings is therefore often misleading. An exploration of manual workers' lifetime earnings would indicate that, while they can go through periods of relative affluence, at other times – family building, bouts of sickness or unemployment, retirement – they may well be prone to poverty. *Figure 1* illustrates this life cycle of poverty.

Figure 1 also indicates that many more people experience poverty than are in it at any one time, the figures for which can therefore be seen as a vast underestimate of the extent of poverty.

Two important points are worth emphasizing, however. Firstly, the incomes of many lower paid white-collar employees are below those of the better-off sections of the manual working class. Secondly, and most crucially, the discussion of wages and salaries usually concentrates on male earnings. Most of the lower paid workers in both the manual and non-manual groups are women.

It was not only the academic research of Goldthorpe and Lockwood that challenged the embourgeoisement thesis. Murdock (1975) notes that 'By far the most damaging counter to the embourgeoisement thesis has come from the overwhelming evidence of the persistence of marked inequali-

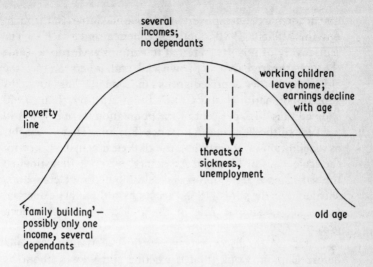

Figure 1 Life cycle of poverty

ties in the distribution of wealth and the rediscovery of family poverty.' He also refers to the subsequent growth in the late 1960s/early 1970s of increased working-class industrial action as the economic situation began to worsen, suggesting that class and class conflict had not disappeared after all.

Further reading

Goldthorpe and Lockwood's study (1969) is still worth looking at. Murdock's (1975) article is interesting for the way it links the myths of classlessness and disappearing poverty to the claim that the 'generation gap' was replacing class as the main social division in society.

The rediscovery of poverty

Despite the optimistic assumptions made in popular, political, and academic debate, poverty had continued to exist through-out the affluent 1950s, both in America and the UK. The rediscovery of poverty, referred to earlier by Murdock, came through the research of Townsend and others among the elderly and other deprived groups in London's East End. His subsequent national study with Brian Abel-Smith in 1960 showed that 14.2 per cent of the population were below 140 per cent of the National Assistance (SB) line. They chose this as a definition of poverty because of their dissatisfaction with the scale rates of National Assistance, which underestimated the subsistence let alone social/cultural needs of claimants. Michael Harrington's (1963) account of 'the other America' performed a similar role in the rediscovery of American poverty.

To talk of a rediscovery suggests the situation of Australia before Captain Cook, that is existing and known about by those in it but not by others. If poverty is seen not to exist then it does not become the basis of social policy since people act on the basis of their definition of the situation, to paraphrase W. I. Thomas; see page 14. There are of course differences between poverty and Australia! One of the many is that Australia does exist in its own right whereas, in a sense, poverty does not – it is a definition of a state of affairs according to a given view or concept of poverty. Sociologists can and do argue over such concepts; they also, on the basis of a given concept of poverty, seek to measure the numbers of people in poverty. Different definitions of poverty will give different measures of the extent of poverty.

Activity

The *Poor Britain* survey (Mack and Lansley 1985) gave people a list of items about such matters as diet, housing, and lifestyle and asked whether they saw these items as necessary or merely desirable for life in the 1980s. The researchers used these answers for their definition of poverty.

Find out what came out of the survey as being necessities. Do you agree with this definition? Are there others you would have included? Give your reasons.

Alternatively you could repeat the survey on a small scale yourselves. You should analyse your results against the social composition of the group you interview.

Getting poverty recognized and responded to is not just a question of publishing sociology books, though sociologists' writings and activities have had an influence on government social policy. Some such writers have been active through the Fabian Society in trying to influence Labour Party social policy. In Britain, in the 1960s, the question of housing shortage was 'popularized' by the television documentary *Cathy Come Home* with the subsequent setting up of Shelter, a campaign and pressure group for the homeless. Later in that decade the Child Poverty Action Group was set up by a group of academics, social workers, and other professionals, committed to welfare reforms to deal with the family poverty to which the growing evidence was pointing.

These few comments on political and pressure group activity indicate the distinction between manifest and latent social problems. Conditions, such as homelessness or malnutrition, can exist for years but remain hidden or unrecognized by those with power or influence, not even defined as social problems at all. These can be seen as latent social problems. A problem may become manifest through the activities of those who are poor or homeless, or those who are concerned about this.

Pressure groups and the media can be important in putting an issue on the political agenda but being on the agenda is not the same as being dealt with satisfactorily. There is widespread acceptance of the view that poverty is a social problem, at least for those seen as the deserving poor, such as the elderly; but, despite the efforts of pressure groups and reformers, it is not diminishing. Marxists tend to argue that this is because the problem of poverty cannot be separated from the problem of capitalist inequality and that 'mere reforms' are not enough; see pages 104 to 113 for more detail on this perspective.

Further reading

The rediscovery of poverty is dealt with by Coates and Silburn (1970). For an account by the former director of the Child Poverty Action Group on its role as a pressure group in the politics of poverty in the 1970s, see Field (1982).

Poverty rediscovered – policy responses

We need to look now at the policy responses by government to the accumulation of evidence that poverty was not disappearing as had been confidently assumed. This discussion will be centred around two themes: the emphasis on community action and projects, especially in the US but in the UK also; the increasing trend in Britain towards greater reliance on means-tested benefits.

Community action in America   After growing awareness and concern in the 1950s about urban decay and its possible link with juvenile delinquency, a number of projects were set up to encourage educational and community participation and renewal. Many of these were incorporated into President Kennedy's 1963 declaration of a War on Poverty, under the auspices of the Office of Economic Opportunity.

These schemes aimed at anything from job training to giving the poor a greater say in their communities. As Marris and Rein point out, in so far as they were successful in the latter they began to upset local mayors and councils. These pressurized the Federal Government to peddle more softly. Indeed Kennedy's successor, Lyndon Johnson, who was also allegedly committed to the anti-poverty programme, withdrew his support from the OEO and reportedly accused it 'of being run by "kooks and sociologists"' – and probably did not intend any distinction between them (Marris and Rein 1974). OEO officials were seen as too ideological and impractical.

With no support from the President, who was becoming increasingly focused on the Vietnam War, they became extremely vulnerable to criticism and they were blamed by some for stirring up the urban riots of summer 1966. In fact, however, as a result of the earlier criticism, the OEO had become more and more cautious and had begun to lose credibility amongst radicals. Thus, as it sought to respond to one set of criticisms, it became more vulnerable to others; just one of the dilemmas noted by Marris and Rein, dilemmas which undermined the programme's chances of success from the very beginning.

Townsend (1976) has linked this policy response to the prevailing theories of poverty in America at the time. He isolates three:

– from orthodox economic theory comes the view which sees poverty in terms of inadequate skills to compete in the labour market;

– from the traditional approach of social work, a stress on the psychological make-up of individuals and families;

– a more sociological view, partly derived from the work of Oscar Lewis (1961), stressed the idea that the poor were trapped in their own poverty by their own way of life. This allegedly stable culture, passed from generation to generation, was centred around fatalism, lack of drive or ambition, and a tendency to only marginal involvement in mainstream social institutions, such as education, trade unionism, politics.

To some degree or another, the poor or their families and communities are blamed for their own poverty. These explanations do not look to the structural causes of poverty, such as in employment, taxation and benefit levels, or the distribution of income, wealth, and power.

The policies resulting from these three theories of poverty were all attempts to break into the so-called culture of poverty or cycle of deprivation. Firstly, there were the job opportunity programmes for unemployed blacks. These did give opportunities to some but overall opportunities were not increased so they simply gave jobs to some at the expense of others.

Secondly, there was some intensive casework with families but this was often resented and 'to a large number of poor people an individualistic explanation of poverty seemed to be more like an ideology of social control'. In other words, if people can be made to feel that their poverty is the product of their own personalities or relationships, then the political and economic structure of society does not get the blame.

Townsend is not saying that these social workers are part of a plot or conspiracy against the poor. What he is saying is that social work practice is too often based on a theory which seeks to explain poverty and other social problems by reference to psychological rather than social factors. Berger (1966) argues that this partly derives from the greater status of psychology in the American popular imagination:

'Social workers have had to fight an uphill battle for a long time to be recognized as "professionals" and to get the prestige, power and (not least) pay that such recognition entails. Looking round for a "professional" model to emulate, they found that of the psychiatrist to be the most natural.'

Whilst this explanation of the casework, clinical interview approach in American (and British?) social work may be rather sketchy, it does point to the possibility that social policy developments can be affected by the interests of welfare professionals and bureaucrats as well as the people they are officially designed to serve.

Thirdly, there were the community action schemes encouraging the poor to organize – as parents, tenants, or such – to demand better services and more resources. As Marris and Rein point out, when these were effective they threatened the local council's power and were squashed or taken over.

Community focus in Britain In Britain there were smaller but still significant attempts to focus the anti-poverty programme on community or local provision. The most notable were: the Plowden Report (1967) on primary schools with its setting up of Educational Priority Areas giving extra resources to schools in those areas; Urban Aid programmes from the late 1960s onwards giving money for nurseries, community centres, and so on; Community Development Programmes whose activities were often quite radical and threatening – they were closed down. In general, says Townsend, these programmes got little money and their effects 'have been only marginal and may have been diversionary'.

One major reason why a poverty programme that concentrates on specific deprived areas is likely to fail is to be found in the wide geographical dispersal of the poor. Retirement pensioners, one parent families, the chronic sick and disabled, and the low paid are not all located in poor inner city areas. Poor though these areas are, poverty can only be tackled by national policies, says Townsend. He points to the importance of attempts to influence the location of industry and employment, of progressive rather than regressive taxation policy, of benefit levels and policies designed to reduce the inequality in wage and salary levels.

Means-tested benefits Beveridge had hoped that National Insurance would be the main plank of the poverty programme. In fact, NI benefit levels were set too low for this task and, over the years, their relative value declined still further. He also hoped that National Assistance with its means test and sense of charity and stigma would be a safety net only used by a few. In 1948, just over one million people were on NA; in the next thirty years, however, this number trebled and has since risen rapidly again.

In addition to their own provision, central government began increasingly to oblige or enable local councils to set up a range of means-tested welfare benefits. The 1944 Education Act had already empowered them to pay allowances to poor

73

parents whose children were staying on at school and to provide school uniform grants for secondary school children. These had little impact. Townsend (1976) has reported huge variations in the generosity of these schemes as well as the massive under-claiming (low take-up) by those with incomes low enough to qualify.

More important in financial terms were the introduction in 1966 of Rate Rebates for low income tenants or owner occupiers and the extension, in 1972, of the rent rebate scheme from council tenants to cover private tenants as well. This provision was merged in 1982/3 to become Housing Benefit. Mortgage payers get tax relief regardless of their income.

In 1970, Family Income Supplement was introduced for those in full-time work, and therefore not entitled to Supplementary Benefit, but whose wages were below the poverty line.

Means-tested benefits are based on a residual approach to social welfare (see page 36) and those who support them argue that, by insisting benefit is dependent on a test of income and circumstances, it concentrates help on the really needy. In doing this it keeps down government spending and therefore taxation. Means-tested benefits are therefore favoured by parties and pressure groups representative of business and the middle classes.

Opponents of means-tested benefits, such as Townsend, argue that they have failed to reduce poverty and are socially divisive by diminishing the status of the poor. Claiming benefits and undergoing a potentially humiliating interview can sometimes act as a process of labelling and self redefinition: 'I am poor, I am a claimant, I am on the welfare.' These self images are at odds with the belief system of a society that values wealth and material success.

More particularly, means-tested benefits are criticized by Bradshaw (1985) who argues that they are complicated and costly to run; that many people do not claim them; and that they create and sustain a poverty trap. The poverty trap is where a person who is claiming benefit receives a wage rise but becomes no better off because they have crossed the qualifying threshold of the benefits involved. Occasionally a person can become worse off after a wage rise because of the loss of benefits.

The take-up rate for benefits has not increased over time as it might have done if it was their newness which was causing the low take-up. *Table 2*, from Bradshaw, provides a range of ways of measuring the extent of take-up for Supplementary Benefit.

Table 2 *Estimates of take-up of Supplementary Benefit (including certificated housing benefit) for 1983*

	nos in receipt (000s)	numbers eligible and not in receipt (000s)	average weekly amount unclaimed £	estimated benefit unclaimed £millions p.a.
pensioners	1,600	790	5.66	233
sick & disabled	200	99	16.28	84
unemployed	1,900	630	22.19	730
one-parent families	430	59	17.32	53
other	170	57	20.50	61
total	4,300	1,640	13.61	1,161

Source: Bradshaw (1985), based on Hansard, House of Commons 1983.

Activity

In Table 2, which groups are proportionately most likely to be eligible for benefit but not claiming it?

How does this fit in with media images of welfare claimants? (See pages 86 to 88).

Many other benefits have a much lower rate of take-up than Supplementary Benefit. Family Income Supplement, for example, after thirteen years of existence still had only half of those entitled actually claiming. In 1983, the combined unclaimed amount of Supplementary Benefit, Family Income Supplement and Housing Benefit was nearly £2 billion.

Further reading

Up to date information on benefit levels, take-up, and so on can be found in the Child Poverty Action Group book edited by Sue Ward (1985), or from other CPAG literature.

Convergence theory and the end of ideology?

End of ideology

This section looks at the claim that the alleged decline in inequality and class was eroding or had eroded the importance of ideological differences within and between societies. Fascism and Nazism had been defeated by World War Two and the full employment of post-war Europe was, it was hoped, an insurance against its revival. Laissez-faire had declined with the apparent acceptance of social and economic management by the state. Socialism was said to be out of date and in decline, as its natural supporters, the working class, were supposedly fast disappearing into the middle class. Feminism was also going through a relatively quiet period in the 1940s and 1950s. It was therefore thought that, not only was there a consensus in social, economic, and political matters, but also ideologcal differences should be seen as a thing of the past.

The main sociological proponent of this view was Daniel Bell (1961) but it was far more than a sociological theory. It became the conventional wisdom of the day, reflected in academic debate and 'common sense' views of the world. In

Britain, the term 'Butskellism' was constructed from the names of Butler and Gaitskell, leading figures in the Conservative and Labour Parties respectively, to denote this consensus view of politics.

The discipline of social administration also reflected this consensus view of the world. With some exceptions, notably that of Titmuss, it had largely become an uncritical subject, concentrating on describing the public welfare activities of government. It tended to see welfare in almost exclusively benevolent terms, not looking at how it can act as a form of social control or questioning its part in reinforcing the conventional roles of women as wives, mothers, and dependants. See the sections on Marxism and feminism for an elaboration on this.

Clearly the 1950s were a period of relative social peace compared to the previous decades. However, the evidence above on continued poverty and inequality, the growth of industrial conflict and the political unrest in the 1960s, associated with racial inequality, the Vietnam War, and student protest, showed it was too soon to pronounce the end of ideology. It is probably more accurate to see that pronouncement as an ideology, in effect asserting that Western societies were progressing happily along a path of 'tamed' or reformed capitalism and that alternatives to this were neither desirable nor feasible. This path of reform and Keynesian economic management has since been criticized by politicians of the New Right (Thatcher, Reagan) as well as from the Marxist left.

Convergence theory

Convergence theory can be seen as a variant on the end-of-ideology thesis and it asserts that, whatever the differences between advanced industrial societies – capitalist or communist – these will diminish as industrialism advances. In the early stages of industrialization, welfare is seen as a functional response to the transition to waged employment, the decline of traditional support systems such as kinship, the growth of urban problems, and, later, the need for an educated and skilled workforce. The speed and nature of this process is determined by the industrializing elite; this was seen in our earlier discussion of the US, Britain and Germany. Later, it is argued, the demands of technology and industrialism begin to shape the nature of society, and the pattern of industrial ownership and ideology becomes less important, though its influence never actually completely disappears.

As a result of this alleged 'logic of industrialism' the state in both capitalist and communist societies comes to play an increasing role in social planning and co-ordination, in education, and in dealing with the health requirements of society. In short, welfare states are functional necessities of advanced industrial societies. Like much functionalist theory, it suggests therefore that things occur because they are necessary or functional to all of society. Critics argue that this overlooks the fact that the needs of many individuals and groups are not met and that welfare developments are often more in the interests of one group or class than another. Mishra (1981) argued that what convergence has occurred between societies is at a very general level and that the theory overlooks enormous differences in levels of coverage and benefits, patterns of taxation and funding, and so on.

The theory lost popularity in the 1960s for the same reasons as the end-of-ideology argument. It was attacked in particular by Marxists who argue that the very use of the term 'industrial society' is misleading for its emphasis on the technological level of the societies in question rather than their political and economic structures, such as who owns industry, who controls the state, and so on. In short, they stress the separateness of capitalism and socialism rather than what they have in common.

Welfare state or capitalist state?

Finally, we need to relate the post-war development of

78

welfare provision to the wider question of the distribution of political power. The Marxist theory of power argues that, by its ownership and control of industry, the capitalist class is able to exert its dominance over state and society. This theory of political power sees the state as primarily acting in the interests of one class, the capitalist or ruling class. This theory is examined in far more detail in the next chapter. Here our concern is with those theories of power which became popular in the 1950s and which asserted that the capitalist class is no longer the ruling class of society, if it ever was. The extension of state and corporate involvement in welfare provision is cited as evidence that the state, and indeed the capitalist class, can and does act for the general good.

There are two variants of this argument: pluralism and managerialism.

Pluralism

Pluralism argues that power, rather than being concentrated in the hands of one class, is spread out among many interests and pressure groups; no group or set of groups is permanently able to dominate. Pressure group activity is seen as the main way that 'the mass of the citizenry brings influence to bear on the decision makers they have elected' (McKenzie 1976).

Pluralism does not see the state as inevitably tied to the interests of one class; it sees it as a neutral institution which can be pushed in various directions by pressure group activity. In this sense, it is based on a functionalist theory of the state which sees the state's power as a collective resource to pursue those common and agreed goals of society that individuals cannot readily or adequately pursue on their own, such as public health and sanitation. As we have seen, pages 46 to 47, some functionalists believe in a minimal role for the state whilst others accept a growing role for government in promoting social solidarity through social and economic policies.

In a sense, pressure group activity is a part by-product of

the welfare state and the growth of state responsibility for disposing of the national income, through taxes and public spending. As the state does more so people want to influence this activity. In another sense, pluralists would point to the welfare state as proof that the state can and does respond to its citizens' needs and demands and, therefore, the welfare state is partly a product of pressure group activity.

Critics do not deny that pressure groups have grown in significance or that they are sometimes successful in pursuing their cases: what they do generally argue is that middle- and upper-class citizens are far more represented than working-class or poor ones. They also point to the major role of institutional pressure groups, such as big business, the mass media, the judiciary, the military, and so on, which would reinforce this class bias. This bias may not be present just in a debate over a particular issue but also in managing to affect what issues get on the agenda. See page 17 for a definition of agenda setting and pages 86 to 88 for an illustration of the role of the press in putting social security fraud rather than tax evasion on the agenda for public and political debate in the mid 1970s.

It should also be noted that many institutions which are not overtly pressure groups on a particular topic may nonetheless have a big stake and influence in such policies. Thus, in the 1985 Social Security Reviews, there were no representatives on the review teams from trade unions or the Child Poverty Action Group but there were two insurance company representatives and two directors of large companies, both also members of the Institute of Directors. The Institute of Directors was also one of the major groups giving evidence to these inquiries. The reviews themselves are dealt with in more detail in the last chapter.

Managerialism

While pluralism holds that the ruling class theory of the state is no longer appropriate because power is now dispersed, another theory which came to the fore in the post-war period argued that the capitalist class was, in any case, undergoing a process of decomposition. This theory, advocated by such writers as Crosland (1956) and Galbraith (1967), starts from the growth in size of companies and corporations and the rise of joint-stock rather than personal ownership of these. These writers argue that with this there has been a separation of ownership and control: there are managers who do not own and owners (shareholders) who do not manage. One version of this theory of managerialism goes on to argue that managers will pursue different company goals to 'old-fashioned' capitalists; they will be socially responsible rather than profit-oriented. Two American writers spoke of the corporation in terms comparable to how pluralists see the state, talking of a 'purely neutral technocracy, balancing a variety of claims by various groups in the community and assigning to each a portion of the income stream on the basis of public policy rather than private cupidity' (Berle and Means 1932). Another American business theorist claimed that 'the modern corporation is a soulful corporation' (Kaysen 1957).

Clearly these arguments are ideological in the sense that they seek or act to defend the growth in size and power of big corporations from the criticism that this is excessive or used only for private gain. It is interesting to note that Berle and Means were writing in the peak years of the American depression when American capitalism was manifestly failing to deliver the goods and American values were so under threat. Today many big companies and multi-nationals are accused of damaging the environment or exploiting the Third World; they are thus acutely aware of their public image.

Activity

From watching commercial television or an analysis of newspaper advertisements, for example in *The Times*, write a list of those adverts which are more concerned with corporate

image than a specific product. What do you think the companies are trying to do by this advertising? To what extent is it an advert for capitalism itself?

On a factual level, managerialist theories point to the growth of occupational or company welfare which occurred rapidly from the 1940s onwards. We have already seen, however, that this growth was patchy and selective, tending to reinforce existing hierarchies of class, income, and gender. General criticisms of the managerialist thesis have argued that managers are usually shareholders or otherwise wealthy and thus their interests and values are not likely to be that distinct from those of owner-managers. For these and other reasons Nichols (1967) argued that rather than talk of a divorce of ownership and control, it is more useful to talk of a marriage of convenience.

Further criticism of managerialism comes from those such as Marxists who claim that managers are not free to pursue goals which conflict with profit-seeking since, under capitalism, profit is the basis of company survival. Marx's critique of capitalism was not founded on the 'greed' or 'nastiness' of capitalists but on the basis that economic demand rather than human need or welfare determined what that society produced. For example, in the early 1970s property developers ('speculators'?) and builders in London were constructing office blocks, often to stand empty for years, rather than decent but reasonably priced housing for the poor. This was not *because* they liked offices and despised the poor, though they may have done. It was because there was profit in the former but not in the latter; there is a difference between wanting a decent home and having the resources to express that desire as demand in the market place.

There are also many examples of owner-managed firms introducing worker welfare schemes, such as that of Rowntree the chocolate maker and poverty researcher who introduced works canteens, sports facilities, personnel management, bonus schemes, and profit sharing. He is quoted as saying that improving workers' conditions is an employer's duty but one which 'does not conflict with his business interests . . . since it is obvious that workers who are in good health and are provided with the amenities of life are more efficient workers' (Kincaid 1975). Blackburn (1965) sees the 1950s/1960s growth of such schemes as a response to trade union pressure, increased productivity and the shortage of skilled labour. Thus, 'A multiplicity of fringe benefits and welfare schemes can become a market necessity, a device for tying the skilled worker to a particular factory.' This latter analysis can be linked to increasing polarization of employment into primary and secondary sectors, discussed on pages 61–2, with primary sector employees reaping the benefit of their stronger position in the labour market.

Conclusion

From the above analysis we can see that the welfare state, along with other social changes, was viewed by many commentators as being associated with a significant decline in inequalities of income, wealth, and power. From the 1960s onwards, many of these arguments and assumptions were challenged, either by research evidence or by increased social conflict and economic recession.

Further reading

Westergaard and Resler (1975) provide a thorough background to many of the above arguments whilst Coates and Silburn (1970) and Field (1981) focus more directly on poverty and social security.

6

Welfare crisis?

In the last chapter, we saw that by the 1960s it was clear that the post-war boom and growth in state welfare provision had neither abolished poverty nor brought about a significant redistribution of income and wealth from rich to poor. This led some commentators to become disillusioned with the welfare state. The slowing down of economic growth in the 1970s led to further pessimism about and criticism of state welfare provision. The economic recession and mass unemployment of the later 1970s and 1980s was associated with shifts in political thinking about welfare. For an indication of the extent of this rise in unemployment, see page 37. Conflict over the welfare state grew, as did the number of cuts in welfare provision, leading many to talk of a welfare crisis.

This section explores the background to this situation and outlines the way writers from the subjects of sociology and social administration have responded to it.

Heclo (1981) points to three general approaches in this disillusion with the welfare state, though he tends to see them all as unnecessarily doom-laden and asserts 'the strength of the underlying welfare state commitment'. These approaches concern:

(i) Cost – here the focus is on an alleged runaway public sector requiring more and more taxation, hitting even low income groups; with this there comes a growing reluctance, especially by the middle class, to pay further taxes for this provision.

(ii) Ineffectiveness – in various ways the welfare state is seen not to be achieving its goals. For example, it is said that it benefits its bureaucrats and professionals more than its clients, that client dependency is encouraged, or that resources do not get to those really in need. Illustration of this first example is to be found in Means' (1977) argument that social work has provided employment 'for those who are above factory work but who lack an entrance into the dominant class'. He also refers to the view of Michels that (capitalist) society has stabilized itself by being able to meet the claims of educated people for secure and satisfactory employment.

(iii) Over-regulation – arguments here suggest that welfare bureaucracies have grown so much in size and power that their interference in people's lives signals a shift from democracy to totalitarianism.

Out of this controversy, says Heclo, have grown a number of more theoretical critiques of the welfare state:

(i) A class analysis – this sees the increased spending as a product of the need of the capitalist class to buy the consent of an increasing number of groups disadvantaged by the workings of capitalism. Out of this growth in state spending comes a monetary crisis. Thus, in the view of the American Marxist O'Connor (see Mishra 1981) the capitalist state is caught in a contradiction between the need both to increase and to control public spending and taxation.

(ii) A demand push analysis – this sees the dilemma in terms of the state having to meet the welfare demands of increasingly well-organized pressure groups for the disadvantaged, often reflecting their large numbers in the electorate.

85

This revolution of rising expectations is said to lead to a growth in demand that just cannot be met.

(iii) A supply push analysis focusing on the way that welfare professionals are able constantly to expand definitions of need and amplify the part of the welfare state in meeting this. The argument for a relative definition of poverty measurement would be seen as part of this process; see page 68 for a definition of relative poverty.

The last two sets of arguments fit very much into what Titmuss (1958) has called the public burden model of welfare and are behind much of the backlash against the welfare state from political groups on the right of the political spectrum.

Politics, the media, and the welfare backlash

Looking in more detail at the development of this welfare backlash, Golding and Middleton (1982) point to how the economic slump of the mid-1970s put welfare at the centre of the political stage. In this, the central issue was not seen to be the problem of poverty and its growth but the cost of welfare and its increase. They note that this concern was international in nature:

– in the Australian General Election campaign, Labour was accused of being soft on so-called welfare cheats and the press talked of 'dole dollies'.

– in Canada, where unemployment was the highest since the 1930s, the press called for attacks on alleged welfare abuse.

– in the US, campaigns for tax cuts and for cuts in services began to surface and the newly elected President Reagan said 'the war on poverty has been won except for a few mopping-up operations'.

– in a number of European countries, parties of the right began to stress anti-welfare/pro-tax cut policies.

Many of these attitudes stem from images and ideologies of welfare and poverty going far into the past and which are discussed in earlier chapters of this book. Golding and

Middleton carried out systematic research into the role of the mass media in focusing and amplifying public anxieties about the recession and unemployment and link their findings to these historical attitudes and prejudices.

'Scrounging' – case study of a moral panic

This research leads them to refer to the growth in political and press concern with alleged welfare abuse as a 'moral panic'. This is a circumstance where a social group or activity is seen as a threat to society's interests or values and is usually given a highly stylized and stereotypical treatment in the media. They locate three stages in the development of this moral panic:

(i) The precipitating event – in this case, the massive publicity given to a Mr Deevy, labelled King Con, found guilty of social security fraud. Great play was made of his cigars and life of luxury.

(ii) The 'discovery' of other supporting stories, reinforcing the implications drawn from the first case. In 1976 the press seemed obsessed with the pursuit of such stories.

(iii) The reaction, such as the employment of extra social security fraud investigators, labelled 'snoopers' by their opponents. This was often reported in warlike terminology, such as 'army of dole cheats'.

The researchers note how the focus shifted from concern with criminal abuse, the cases of which were always seen as the tip of the iceberg, to a concern about welfare in general. Social security was seen as too generous, too easy to get, too readily abused and too complex in administration. The reporting of this often drew upon other negative stereotypes of the 'undeserving' poor – the 'lazy' unemployed or 'immoral' single mothers who came increasingly under official suspicion – or was linked to hostility to black people, usually defined as immigrants. These groups became defined in the press as outsiders and they were contrasted with the 'good honest citizens and taxpayers'. The question of taxpayers is interesting, for Novak (1984) points out that

'In 1979, the 5,000 and more officials employed by the DHSS to police the social security system prosecuted 29,000 claimants, most of them for small amounts. In contrast, the Inland Revenue employed only 260 investigators and prosecuted 184 tax defrauders.'

A House of Commons Public Accounts Committee report on Schedule D tax returns from the self-employed showed that in 1982, of those investigated, 87.3 per cent had underpaid.

It is worth noting that general evidence of social security fraud was difficult to find. The 1973 Fisher Committee on Abuse of Social Security Benefits found less than 1 per cent of all claims involved abuse. We have already noted on pages 74 to 76 the very large sums that go unclaimed every year in social security benefits of various kinds. The fact that many papers lack a welfare correspondent and rely on crime reporters picking up social security fraud stories at court partly accounts for the focus on criminal abuse.

Further reading

Golding and Middleton summarised some of their research findings in New Society, 26 October, 1978. Barrat (1986) *places the debate in the context of the sociology of the mass media.*

Wages, benefits, and poverty

The claim that social security benefits are too high is an interesting one. It can be seen to revolve around two issues. Firstly, there is the question of the definition of poverty. Those who see social security benefits as too high often deny the existence of poverty or 'real' poverty, usually defined in absolute terms and geared to mere physical survival or in terms of images of squalor and deprivation derived from pre-war Britain. Evidence from the 'Poor Britain' survey (Mack and Lansley 1985) shows that such deprivation still exists. Clearly, however, if we recall the life cycle of poverty described in the last chapter, it will be seen that, by the time some people's incomes fall below the poverty line, they may already have a well-furnished home with a television and so on. Thus whilst their poverty may be invisible to others, their income may still be barely enough to subsist on, let alone anything else. In general, the absolute condition of the poor has improved over the post-war period but, in relation to average earnings, social security benefits have not significantly improved since the Beveridge package was implemented (Field 1981). Those who adopt a relative definition of poverty, such as Townsend (1979), argue that benefit levels need upgrading considerably.

From this, it will be obvious that the kind of poverty definition a person adopts is neither random nor purely a question of academic argument. It is inevitably linked to their view of society and political persuasion.

The second issue in the debate reflects back to the 1834 principle of less eligibility. In its modern form this argues that benefit levels should not be high enough to discourage the unemployed from working, even at a low paid job. It became almost conventional wisdom in the mid-1970s that many people were better off on the dole than in work and that, as a result, a large portion of unemployment was self-imposed. The ideological function of such a claim is to divert attention away from causes of unemployment that relate to the workings of the capitalist economy or the policies pursued by government. Golding and Middleton (1978) point out that the problem was always defined in terms of high benefits rather than low wages. The DHSS report, *Social Assistance* (1978), showed that only with four or more children would a man on the dole receive more than 90 per cent of his income while working. Significantly, in terms of the traditional view of the unemployed as undeserving, they can never qualify for the long term rate of Supplementary Benefit, introduced in 1966 and now about 20 per cent higher than ordinary scale rates. In May 1977, 16 per cent of the unemployed received no benefit at all, either National Insurance or Supplementary Benefit.

As unemployment levels rose by over two million in the years 1979 to 1983 and stabilized at between three and five million, depending on the method of calculation, the focus on benefit levels as an alleged cause of unemployment seemed to subside. A new theory of self-inflicted unemployment began to surface however. It was argued by government ministers and others that workers were pricing themselves out of jobs.

Many free market theorists suggested abolishing Wages Councils, the statutory bodies laying down minimum rates in low wage industries, so that wages could find their own level, that is, fall. Opposition to this appeared too strong, though it was announced on the 17 July, 1985 that 500,000 workers under twenty-one in industries covered by the Councils will from 1986 cease to benefit from their protection. Research by the Low Pay Unit has shown that illegal underpaying by employers is growing and research in Greater Manchester showed that, in 1984, 43 per cent of the sample of the county's employers who were visited by government wages inspectors were found to be illegally underpaying all or some of their staff (*Guardian* 7 May, 1985). There have been allegations that the government has encouraged these inspectors to turn a blind eye to such underpaying. Whether this is true or not, the contrast between government treatment of fraudulent social security claimants and employers illegally underpaying workers seems quite massive. This illustrates one of the major themes in the sociology of crime and deviance, namely that power or its absence has a great deal to do with one's chance of being prosecuted or having one's activities defined as criminal.

90

Further reading

Mack and Lansley (1985) is an excellent up-to-date survey of poverty, attitudes to poverty, and the debate about how to define it; four one-hour television programmes were based on it and are available in video from Breadline Britain, Educational Cassette, Box 33, London SE1 9LT.

Poor Law by Roz Franey (1983) gives a detailed discussion of 'Operation Major', a police/DHSS swoop on social security fraud in Oxford, and shows the massive official (over)reaction to this issue.

Conclusion

By the mid-1970s, then, it was clear that whatever consensus on welfare provision had existed was fast disappearing. One of the last examples of Parliamentary consensus on welfare matters was Labour's 1975 social security Pensions Act introducing the State Earnings Related Pension Scheme, to come into force in 1978. This provided for an earnings-related additional pension on top of the basic flat rate provision and would be based on the best twenty years of a person's working life, a scheme favourable to women workers whose interrupted pattern of earnings might disadvantage them on any scheme based on the last twenty years of earnings. The scheme was to be guaranteed against inflation by the government and, a new provision, either spouse could inherit their dead partner's pension rights. Those with satisfactory private occupational schemes could opt out of the scheme. The 1985 Conservative Green Paper on the future of the social security system proposed to abolish SERPS (as it is known), but opposition forced them to back down; instead its value is to be significantly reduced.

The criticisms of welfare provision that gained most prominence in the media were those of the political right, though alternative critiques were also being put forward. Marxists and feminists were increasingly pointing to the repressive and ideological role of state welfare as well as its failure or inability to break down inequalities of class and gender. Within the discipline of social administration itself, there was a growing recognition of the conflicting ideologies and perspectives on welfare provision. One of the first and most significant analyses was that of George and Wilding (1976).

Welfare perspectives

It was common in the 1950s, both in the academic discipline of social administration and much political debate, to see welfare as 'a good thing' and more of it as even better. Welfare criticism tended to focus on gaps or inefficiencies in welfare provision. George and Wilding's analysis demonstrates a more complex range of approaches to welfare, based on different or even contradictory social values and views of society. They distinguish four ideological groupings, categorized largely in terms of their attitude to state welfare provision. All four are briefly outlined below. Two of them – the reluctant collectivists and the Fabians – were significant in shaping the wartime welfare consensus and the 1950s consensus approach to party politics. In that sense, they have been quite fully explored already though a more systematic outline of their key beliefs is now called for. The other two perspectives – Marxism and the anti-collectivists/New Right – are given much fuller treatments in later sections. The four are:

(i) The anti-collectivists, who see state welfare as unnecessary and undesirable since the individual can and should provide for himself through the market by what he earns or buys, including private health, pension, or insurance. Recently these views have been vigorously advocated by supporters of what is called the New Right; see pages 96 to 104.

(ii) The reluctant collectivists, who value individual effort and self-help but see state action as necessary to counter the effects of economic slumps and other flaws in the workings of the capitalist market economy.

(iii) The Fabian socialists, who welcome state welfare provision as necessary and desirable; they see it as a move towards a more just society and even as a step on the road to socialism.

(iv) Marxists, who are largely but not completely critical of what they see as the generally limited value of the social reforms or their role in boosting or reinforcing capitalism by building up the strength of workers or buying off discontent; see pages 104 to 113.

The reluctant collectivists

As exponents of this approach, George and Wilding chose Keynes and Beveridge from the UK and the American economist Galbraith. What they have in common is a general belief in individual liberty and the system of free enterprise (capitalism). They do accept, however, that poverty and extreme inequality restrict personal liberty and that, therefore, some social and economic action by the government is necessary. This is reinforced by their view that capitalism without government economic and social planning will experience slumps and mass unemployment. These not only cause suffering and loss of freedom but are a waste of resources.

Their attitude to state action, then, is mixed. In general, they would prefer a laissez-faire policy but do not believe it works. Government action is therefore essential and, indeed, potentially benevolent. They do, however, believe that excessive state action can lead to all-powerful government of a totalitarian kind.

There are differences between these writers. Both Keynes and Beveridge see the state in neutral or functionalist terms while Galbraith sees it more in terms of conflict theory, noting how dominant economic interests, mainly big business, have effectively hijacked the state for their own purposes.

Finally, we should note a criticism of the inclusion of Beveridge as a reluctant collectivist. A number of writers have argued that whilst, in his early career, he had a liberal wariness of government action, by the 1940s he had become a thorough-going collectivist.

The Fabian socialists

The main difference between these and the reluctant collectivists is that the former place much greater stress on equality as a goal and are more positive about the value of state action. Fabians differ widely in their own political beliefs, however. Some, such as Tawney, wanted the kind of fundamental reorganization of society called for by Marxists, though they differ from Marxists in that they believe that gradual and peaceful reforms by government can and will lead to a socialist society. Townsend is in this radical tradition of Fabianism. Others, such as Crosland in the 1950s, saw capitalism as already having been tamed and reformed out of all recognition; see pages 59, 65, and 80–1.

The commitment to equality comes from a belief that class inequalities hinder the discovery of talent and thereby waste resources. By denying individual potential and freedom they are also unjust. They further argue that excessive inequality leads to class antagonism and restricts social integration.

Activity

Using any standard textbook on sociology, look up the functionalist theory of stratification of Davis and Moore. Contrast their arguments in favour of inequality with the arguments of the Fabians who see greater equality as functional, rather than inequality.

Fabians place great emphasis on collective goals and social

integration. They reject the morality of the market forces of supply and demand in distributing goods and services as being simply based on the power (wealth) of consumers rather than the needs of individuals. Government intervention or regulation is therefore necessary to limit the impact of market forces. Marxists criticize their approach to this as piecemeal; they are in favour of the complete abolition of market forces.

Citizenship and social welfare One of the writers within the Fabian tradition, T. H. Marshall, is explored in more detail by Mishra (1981) in his somewhat different and rather more directly sociological approach to welfare perspectives.

Marshall distinguished between civil rights (such as equality before the law, freedom from arbitrary arrest), political rights (such as voting or standing for public office), and social rights (concerned with social and economic security). Each is seen as a form of citizenship and the development of the first two in the eighteenth and nineteenth centuries respectively is seen as contributing to the development of the third in the twentieth century. The struggle for social rights is seen as reaching its peak in the Beveridge proposals for universal provision through social insurance, family allowances, and the NHS. As this suggests, it is an approach to welfare based largely on British history and has limited value when applied to other countries. In Germany, for example, Bismarck introduced social insurance as a way of preventing the spread of demands for democratic rights. In the USA, democratic rights (for whites) came earlier than in Britain but social rights much later.

As a perspective on welfare, citizenship can be used as a justification for an institutional approach to welfare, stressing 'as-of-right' benefits rather than a residual and stigmatized means-tested approach (see page 36). The Beveridge Report was sprinkled with references to the importance of citizenship.

The welfare backlash in the 1970s referred to by Golding and Middleton (1978) rejects welfare universalism and has sought to narrow the definition of citizenship by a constant reference to alleged scroungers as distinct from tax-paying 'citizens'. Thus, in their media treatment claimants are accorded a reduced status as citizens. Where claimants are also black, this status is often reduced still further by racist stereotyping in the mass media or by the use of passport checks at DHSS offices. This and other aspects of racism in social security are discussed more fully in Chapter 7.

Further reading

For a wider discussion of racist stereotyping in the mass media, see Barrat (1986).

Harrison's Inside the Inner City *(1983), a valuable though not directly sociological study of deprivation in a London borough, gives a critical view of the role and workings of the social security system in the inner city. It is very readable.*

The New Right

Earlier it was noted that the economic recession of the mid-1970s had led to a welfare backlash amongst some politicians and many sections of the popular press. It was also noted how media criticism of alleged welfare abuse was generalized into a wholesale critique of the system of social welfare. The theoretical basis of this attack is to be found in the writings of the academics and politicians of the New Right. Many of these are committed to the laissez-faire views of such writers as F. Hayek, author of *The Road to Serfdom* (1976, first published in 1944), and grouped by George and Wilding under the heading of the anti-collectivists.

In one sense the New Right is not new at all. This is indicated by the name of one of the leading research organizations and pressure groups for these views, the Adam Smith Institute, named after the eighteenth century economist. It is also shown by the frequent positive references by right-wing Conservative politicians to a selection of Victorian values. For example, a former Conservative Social Security Minister, Rhodes Boyson, refers to the self-help of the Victorian era, with 'its virtues of duty, order and efficiency' when 'religious responsibility and individual conscience ensured that profits and wealth were seen as a trust to be spent aright' (1971).

In another sense, however, the New Right is a radical departure from the post-war consensus on matters of economics and welfare. Whilst one writer for the Institute of Economic Affairs, a right-wing pressure group, had argued in 1961 that 'the true object of the Welfare State . . . is to teach people how to do without it' (quoted in Clarke 1983), the real impact of the New Right is very definitely of the 1970s and 1980s. This can be indicated by one mainstream account of the welfare state published in 1980. Its author, David Marsh, was able to claim that today 'we no longer have . . . arguments about the need for the state to plan economic and social policies'. He also argued that there are

> 'certainly no major political groups, who publicly advocate that the coal, electricity, gas, and even railway industries should be taken out of the hands of the state; that the Post Office, the Bank of England, the BBC, British Airways, Cable and Wireless Ltd., and the crown lands should be handed over to private enterprise.'

> (Marsh 1980)

Five years later the following are being or are already privatized: BA, British Gas, Cable and Wireless, and, of course, British Telecom.

The policies of the New Right were first espoused in government in Britain by Mrs Thatcher in 1979 and in the US by Mr Reagan a year later. What are the values of these new anti-collectivists?

97

Values

According to George and Wilding (1976), the three main values of the anti-collectivists are:

(i) A stress on the liberty of the individual, particularly in relation to economic activity. This leads them to oppose the organized power of interest groups, though Armstrong, Glyn, and Harrison (1984) argue that in practice it is the power of organized labour through trade unions that has been most opposed.

(ii) A stress on voluntary rather than state action in welfare provision (which leads on from point (i)). Hence Boyson's stress on charity and self-help and the general emphasis by the New Right on the role of the family in providing welfare. In their view the state should have only a 'night-watchman' role.

(iii) Inequality: unequal rewards are seen as necessary to the rewarding of success and provide incentives for wealth creation. It is this, rather than the redistribution of wealth, which they see as the key to the abolition of poverty. Taxes on high incomes are seen to undermine effort; in 1971 Boyson claimed that 'the state spends all its energies taking money from the energetic, successful and thrifty to give to the idle, the failures and the feckless.' Sir Keith Joseph, another Conservative minister, argued that government action in pursuit of equality can only take place at the expense of freedom and 'will turn this country into a totalitarian slum'. Just as the title of this book is *Whose Welfare?*, we could ask whose freedom will be lost by greater equality of income and wealth.

Activities

1 By referring to the earlier data on taxes and benefits, list the arguments for or against the views of Boyson just outlined.
2 Using a standard sociology textbook:
   (a) compare the justification of inequality here with the

functional theory of stratification as argued by Davis and Moore.

(b) examine the criticisms of this theory put forward by such writers as Tumin (1953). To what extent do they apply to the views of Sir Keith as well?

3 Read the following quotation from Rhodes Boyson's *Down with the Poor*. It is meant to be an account of how the British welfare state operates.

'I recently read about the breeding in America of the first bald chickens. Apparently it seemed obvious to detached observers and researchers, if not to the chickens, that farmers could save much time and money if chickens ceased to have feathers. Valuable food is wasted on the production of feathers and an appalling amount of effort is required to pluck them before the chicken is oven ready. The interests of the chicken would further be served by the elimination of the superfluous feathers since these provide a home for dirty little parasites which make the chicken itch and scratch to ease its discomfort. Compassion as well as economy required the disappearance of the feathers.

'Alas the result was completely different from what was intended. Economically the first 200 bald chickens suffered so severely from the cold that they actually required much more food and warmth than did their feathered brethren. In addition to these economic disincentives the chickens suffered from such a lack of physical and moral fibre that they laid fewer eggs and tended to develop ulcers.'

(a) What claims about the welfare state and its alleged effects are contained in the passage?
(b) How valid do you think the claims are?

Thatcherism and the rise of the New Right in Britain

The break with past attitudes to welfare represented by the New Right was associated with a shift in control of the

Conservative Party. Following Mrs Thatcher's election as Conservative leader in 1975 and then Prime Minister in 1979, the anti-collectivists have come to exert effective domination of the party. In doing this, what might be called Tory paternalism has been pushed to one side.

In this move to dominance, the battle over ideas was crucial. Apart from the influence of the media, the role of research organizations set up to promote right-wing ideas, such as the Central Policy Review Staff (or Think Tank), was important, as were pressures from outside the party from such organizations as the Institute of Directors. The Institute of Directors has been one of the strongest proponents of cuts in state welfare spending over recent years.

The New Right in government – Thatcher and Reagan

As we have seen, one of the main elements of the ideology of the New Right is the classical liberal or laissez-faire view of the state; that is, that the state should intervene as little as possible in the running of society and the economy. Thus Wilding (1983) points to the absence of any significant reference to poverty in the 1979 Conservative General Election manifesto or to policies for combating it. The reasons for this, he says, are a belief that poverty is functional, acting as a deterrent to laziness, and is best escaped by self-help; that social security is too soft already, encouraging dependence on the state, rather than self-reliance; and that more welfare can be achieved through greater efficiency and increased use of the informal sector (charity, voluntary help, the family) rather than the state.

Andrew Gamble (1985) argues that the New Right draws on another ideological tradition as well as the doctrine of the minimal state. The second tradition stresses the importance of order and discipline in society and values a strong state, strengthened power of employers over workers, and a general reassertion of the value of authority and hierarchy. This, says Gamble, explains the paradox of a government committed to a reduced role for the state actually increasing its centralized power, such as in control over local government, and increased emphasis on law and order. Thus, from 1978/79 and 1985/86 spending in real terms on law and order rose by 40 per cent while on housing it fell 51 per cent and on education it remained static. Spending on health and personal social services rose 20 per cent, partly reflecting increased costs of health care and the demands of an ageing poulation. There was a substantial rise in social security spending, also reflecting the increased numbers of elderly as well as of single parents and, more especially, the rise of two million in the numbers officially unemployed.

Gamble also argues that the attempt by the New Right to dismantle the post-war consensus and reorganize society along more laissez-faire and authoritarian lines has often made it more rather than less interventionist. There has been open conflict with traditionally quite conservative institutions, such as the BBC, the universities, and the Church of England. In addition there has been unprecedented intervention in the finances of local government, and the abolition of the GLC and metropolitan councils as well as several rounds of legislation affecting the organization and funding of trade unions and the Labour Party. Firm financial control of nationalized industries has been imposed and they have been forced to keep to tight budgets and profit deadlines. The conflicts in the steel and coal industries are indications of a willingness to confront what are seen as the powerful interest groups of trade unionism. Opposition to state subsidies and vested interests has not been consistent, however, as the following examples indicate:

(i) In 1984 the government backed down over plans to make middle and higher income groups pay towards the university fees of their children.

(ii) In the same year it refused to accept a proposal by a report chaired by the Duke of Edinburgh that mortgage tax relief be abolished. Once again, it seemed the power of the middle class appeared too great.

(iii) Agriculture receives £2 billion a year subsidy from British taxpayers, about £35 for each child, woman, and man. Half of this subsidy goes to the 10,000 biggest farmers, all of them millionaires (*Guardian* 18 February, 1985 and 1 March, 1985).

The results – the social impact of Thatcherism   From the point of view of social security provision, Golding (1983) suggested that the most important impact of Thatcherism had been ideological. By this he meant that it had been able to convert the experiences and anxieties of the public into the language of cuts and welfare burden, of excessive state spending and taxation. The ideology of laissez-faire became expressed as 'common sense'. Since then there have been major reviews of social security provision with possible massive repercussions for the future; these are discussed separately later.

There have been a number of cumulative changes in social security benefits, including those concerning strikers and Supplementary Benefit (see page 108), as well as the abolition of earnings-related sickness and unemployment benefits and the taxing of unemployment benefits. Certain benefits have also been improved, notably Family Income Supplement and one-parent benefit.

Taking into account changes in tax rates and benefits, research from the Institute of Fiscal Studies shows that budget changes from 1978/79 to 1985/86 have left only 6 per cent of the population better off and 87 per cent worse off (*Guardian* 18 July, 1985). This is on top of a significant widening of income inequality before taxes and benefits. From 1979 to 1985 the gross earnings of the top 10 per cent rose by 101 per cent whilst those of the bottom 10 per cent rose by 70 per cent; inflation rose by 75 per cent (New Earnings Survey, *Guardian* 30 October, 1985). The *Poor Britain* survey (Mack and Lansley 1985) found 7 million people below their poverty line in 1984.

The results – America and Reaganism   In Britain, so long as the Prime Minister's party has a majority in the House of Commons, it can usually get its proposals for legislation through Parliament, though not always. In America, the system of government and party organization is different and Presidential proposals may well be defeated by the American Congress. Thus, in 1982, Congress voted 96 to 0 against proposals to cut certain social security and medicare programmes.

In other areas of welfare, President Reagan's New Right policies have brought cuts. In 1981, central government responsibility for welfare and food stamps was reduced (*Sunday Times* 3 February, 1985). Also that year, unemployment benefit was denied to any of the 140,000 who had recently left the army and were eligible for re-enlistment or who had been discharged for bad conduct. States were also encouraged to set up 'workfare' schemes to force unemployed people to join clubs where form-filling, reading job advertisements, and so on were imposed for forty hours a week, or where people were forced to work for the state at a minimum rate of pay (Armstrong, Glyn, and Harrison 1984). A range of benefits will no longer be automatically increased to take inflation into account. By 1983, 35 million Americans were officially below the poverty line, including almost one child in four, a 50 per cent increase on the mid-1960s. The US Census Bureau found that, in 1984, 30 per cent of the US population (66 million) were receiving some kind of welfare benefit, with dependence on means-tested benefits twice as high among black families as whites.

As in the UK, some bishops have come to be concerned at the widening gap between rich and poor. A pastoral letter from the nation's Roman Catholic bishops stated that 'The distribution of income and wealth in the US is so unequal that it violates the minimum standard of distributive justice' (*Observer* 18 November, 1984). The implication of this new criticism is that the inequality, before it was widened by

Reagan, was acceptable, indicating perhaps that the bishops are generally quite conservative on such matters.

As in the UK also, the massive increase in unemployment and a more abrasive stance by government has cut trade union membership and weakened trade union influence. From 1974 to 1984, US union membership dropped by 16 per cent to bring about the smallest proportion of the workforce in trade unions for forty years, only 18 per cent.

One significant difference between the US and the UK is that American provision had gone less far and debate on state welfare was generally more sceptical or hostile. For this reason, Thatcherism can be seen as more of a break with the past than Reaganism and needs to bring about more sweeping social changes to impose its anti-collectivist values on society.

Further reading

Ways of keeping informed on the policies of the New Right in Britain should include regular use of the conservative daily press, especially the Daily Telegraph *or* The Times, *as well as the speeches of Tory MPs, debates at the Conservative Party Conference (held each autumn), and their manifesto for the next general election. See also the material on the social security reviews.*

A critical approach to these policies can be found in the Guardian *and the writings of the Child Poverty Action Group.*

Marxism

Whilst Marxist approaches to social welfare have been met already, the growth in the last two decades of Marxist analyses of welfare now makes a fuller account necessary.

Background ideas

First we need to have some grasp of Marxism itself. Some of the main elements can be summarized as follows:

(i) Societies are best categorized in terms of their economic type or mode of production. Much of the rest of society's organization and belief systems is shaped by this.

(ii) The mode of production includes both the forces of production (land, labour, capital, and so on) and the relations of production (the pattern of ownership and control of the means of production).

(iii) Thus, in terms of the forces of production, Britain is an industrial society but, because its industry is privately owned and run for profit, it is also a capitalist society.

(iv) The division of society into classes based on ownership and non-ownership gives rise to class division and class conflict. The two main classes are the capitalist, and the proletariat or working class; Marx did recognize other class divisions, however.

(v) The proletariat have no means of livelihood apart from the sale of their labour power to a capitalist employer. This leads them into a position of exploitation by the capitalist class giving rise to widespread poverty, deprivation, and massive inequality.

(vi) The workings of the capitalist economy and the power of the capitalist class give that class a dominant position in relation to the state. This dominance means that even a government with a large majority in Parliament is limited in what it can do if it seeks to act against long-term capitalist interests.

(vii) Because of this, the state is seen largely in terms of the part it plays in promoting capitalist interests and keeping the working class in its place.

Marxism and social problems

Following from this, Marxists argue that most of the social

problems of capitalism stem from the capitalist mode of production itself. In other words, it is the unequal distribution of wealth and power and the organization of production for profit which are the sources of exploitation and poverty. As a result, Marxists are usually sceptical of the value of reforms which leave untouched the cause of the problem – the capitalist system itself. For them, nothing short of the abolition of capitalism by revolution can solve these problems, though they do accept the possibility of a peaceful overthrow of capitalism. Nonetheless they do recognize that workers have to live under that system until its replacement by socialism and that they have often, therefore, sought to make improvements in their living and working conditions. Marxists generaly support such struggles and reforms.

A Marxist analysis of welfare reform would therefore tend to point to its potentially contradictory nature. By modifying the workers' exploitation, it may weaken their revolutionary ardour and thereby undermine the chances of a more fundamental change and a 'real' improvement in their conditions.

Marxism, welfare, and social control

An example of the way reforms are seen as limited and even contradictory is shown by Marx's own view of nineteenth century factory reform. Whilst Parliament was pushed into passing such legislation, it did little to enforce it. Much more recent research shows widespread breaches of factory legislation in England but extremely few prosecutions (Carson 1971).

This leniency in the face of business crime as well as in relation to tax evasion is contrasted by Marxists and others with the legal and media persecution of social security abuse or fraud, discussed on pages 86 to 88. The *Observer* (22 December, 1985) reports that social security fraud prosecutions outnumber tax evasion cases by more than fifty to one. They point to the class differentiation in the way the law is enforced or defined as another feature of capitalist inequality. Just as the state is not seen as neutral, neither is law and order.

Kincaid (1975) points to the existence of similar inequality in the concept of 'industrial misconduct' in National Insurance regulations. Where a worker is sacked by his or her employer for industrial misconduct, that person may lose up to six weeks' unemployment benefit. What is interesting is that such an offence can only be committed by a worker, never by an employer. Whilst such a worker would qualify for Supplementary Benefit, a deduction for this offence would be made from the weekly rate; this six-week penalty was raised in 1971 from 75p a week to 40 per cent of the Supplementary Benefit rate for a single person.

Activity

Find out what the current SB rate for a single person is and then work out what the 40 per cent penalty for industrial misconduct would be.

It is worth mentioning also that the National Insurance Commissioner has ruled that hearsay and other evidence which would not be acceptable in an ordinary court is allowable in these cases.

The rule about disqualification and deductions from benefits also applies to those who are deemed to have left their work voluntarily. Kincaid (1975) refers to cases which indicate that leaving a job to avoid being pressurized into joining a trade union was considered reasonable but leaving a non-union firm which did not recognize union rules about work practices was not. In short, he argues that National Insurance decisions tend to be anti-union and pro-employer.

The social control or discipline of the workforce is also enforced through having a large pool of unemployed. This makes workers more easily replaced and thereby weakens trade unions and undermines wage levels. Some theorists, not all of them Marxists, have argued that unemployment has reinforced the trend towards a polarized labour market of primary and secondary workers (see pages 61 to 62). The latter, with poor wages, status, and security, are often made up of women, and black or migrant workers. The strength of the working class is therefore weakened by racial and sexual divisions, with the white, male working class exploited by capitalism but generally gaining at the expense of black and female workers.

Strikes, welfare, and social control – the miners' strike 1984/85
Marxists and other radicals point to the 1984/85 miners' strike as an illustration of the ways in which welfare can be used as a political weapon or a form of social control. Hilary Rose (1985) has placed the strike in the context of the breaking of the 1939–45 compromise or settlement 'in which capital and labour negotiated a bargain which exchanged social rights for social peace'. Many of these rights and benefits have been eroded or withdrawn and the Conservative Government is seen to accept the loss of social peace and the confrontation this brings as a necessary feature of its new social and economic policies.

From the points of view of the strike Rose, as well as Jones and Novak (1985), refers in particular to the 1980 Social Security Acts which introduced the assumption that all strikers receive regular strike pay from their union and made a compulsory deduction from payments to strikers' dependants; this was raised from £15 to £16 a week in November 1984. Strikers themselves receive no Supplementary Benefit payment and the Act withdrew the discretionary power that the DHSS had to make urgent needs payments to single strikers in cases of 'overwhelming necessity'. Thus while strikers' families were forced to live below the poverty line and child benefit became even more important, single strikers had no means of support at all. The Secretary of State, Patrick Jenkin, explained that the Acts were part of a strategy 'to restore a fairer bargaining balance between employers and trade unions', which, say Marxists, means a strategy of weakening the working class and its organizations.

Miners' wives in low paid jobs who sought to claim Family Income Supplement found that their husbands' wages from before the strike and the previous overtime ban were taken into account in refusing them benefit. Miners sacked during the dispute were refused unemployment benefit while the strike lasted and still had the £16 per week Supplementary Benefit deducted from their families' benefit. Conservatives in the House of Lords were calling for stricter investigation on how families spent their benefit, especially those who were receiving money to cover the cost of mortgage interest payments (the DHSS never makes mortgage capital repayments). Many of the changes in benefit practice were contained in a special document on 'additional guidance' for DHSS staff which became public in the third month of the strike.

Outside the Supplementary Benefit system, local authorities have the power to make payments to families under child care legislation where it would prevent family break-up or children being taken into care. These payments were treated by the DHSS as income, whether they were grants or just loans, and deducted from any Supplementary Benefit claim; except for £4 – called a 'disregard'. Meal vouchers for miners' children were treated the same way. Finally, despite advice from the Attorney General that striking miners were entitled to pension credits for the year, the Coal Board was seeking ways to avoid paying them (*Guardian* 9 August, 1985).

The absence of official welfare provision can be seen as a part explanation of the development of unofficial welfare through miners' support groups and, especially, the practical aid organized by the women in the mining communities.

Marxism and welfare explanations

We have already seen that Saville (1957/58), about England, and Piven and Cloward (1972, 1982), about America, stress a mixture of factors in explaining welfare development and only a brief summary is necessary here:

(i) The desire by employers for a healthier and more efficient workforce.

(ii) The recognition by the propertied that some 'ransom' would have to be paid if their privileges were to be preserved.

(iii) The struggle by the working class for improvements in their living standards and working conditions.

These struggles have often been opposed by business interests despite the recognition by some employers that welfare developments need not undermine capitalist interests. The recognition of this is important. The Marxist feminist Elizabeth Wilson (1980) stresses the importance of this fact and criticizes some other Marxists for their tendency to dismiss all welfare reforms as functional to capitalism or even a kind of automatic adjustment of capitalism to threats or stresses.

Marxism and the state

Discussion of Marxist approaches to welfare and social problems centres around their analysis of the state. For Marxists the state is an expression of class domination. They argue that this dominance comes through one or more of the following factors:

(i) The social background of many of the main state elites – politicians, judges, military officers, and top civil servants – gives them a vested interest in hierarchy, property, and privilege. Their family, education, and career socialization is likely to reinforce such values.

(ii) The power of business and related pressure groups. Here the City financial institutions, the Confederation of British Industry, the multi-national corporations, most of the national press, and even the American government are pointed to.

(iii) The limitations placed on anti-capitalist action by the workings of the market itself. Here, for example, the role of profit as the determinant of economic choices under capitalism (in investment decisions, wages policies, and so on) means that profit is essential for national economic well-being but it is also furthering the interests of the capitalist class in particular. Only by replacing the market and profit as the basis of production can this be fully overcome. This is why Mishra (1981) refers to a Marxist's approach to welfare as structural; it involves the wholesale reorganization of society so that need is the determinant of production and distribution.

(iv) The organization of the state, from its constitutional rules to its means of policy formation, is geared to the prevention of major threats to the political and economic organization of society ever becoming seriously entertained.

By these means, then, the state is so constituted as to reinforce the position of the capitalist class. Marxists do accept, however, that the state has some autonomy and can act against business pressure to further the long term interests of the capitalist class or even to concede rights and reforms to the working class.

In more concrete terms, the part the state plays in reinforcing capitalism, says Cockburn (1977), can be divided into its role in reproducing:

(i) The forces of production, including labour power. This might lead it into road building to aid industry, subsidies for investment or research, or the provision of education for a trained workforce.

(ii) The relations of production. Here stress is placed on the ideological and social control role of welfare, ranging from the industrial discipline described above to the part played by teachers, social workers, and health visitors as state regulators of people's behaviour. Many of these are employed by local authorities and for this, and other reasons, Cockburn argues that councils – as local states – must be seen as extensions of the centralized capitalist state.

A somewhat similar distinction is made by O'Connor (in Mishra 1981) who sees the state as seeking to ensure the long term efficiency and profitability of capitalist industry and, secondly, to promote social harmony in order to legitimize the capitalist system. These goals are contradictory, says O'Connor, since the constant increases in government spending for the latter mean the diversion of funds away from profitable areas of economic activity.

A hypothetical example of this is to see the high levels of unemployment as having been introduced in order to lower wages levels and weaken trade unionism. Through this, profitability is increased. However, to reduce the chances of massive social conflict and unrest, unemployment or Supplementary Benefit is paid to these people. This state spending to maintain social stability diverts money away from investment in economically productive areas and therefore contradicts the original goal. This contradiction is seen to be the source of a potential crisis of welfare capitalism.

Marxism and the welfare state

We can now draw together the general analysis above and the earlier discussion of the post-war welfare expansion and suggest the main ingredients of a Marxist approach to the welfare state.

Activity

Before reading the section below, the reader might like to list what some of the main features of a Marxist analysis of the modern British welfare state might be.

(i) The term 'welfare state' is misleading since it implies a benevolent state rather than one which acts to maintain class domination and inequality.

(ii) The reforms associated with the welfare state were important gains for the deprived and working class.

(iii) These reforms have not, however, even abolished poverty let alone significantly reduced the inequality in the distribution of income and wealth. This is particularly the case when the tax allowance welfare state is taken into consideration. Much of the welfare state redistribution has been of a horizontal, rather than vertical, kind.

(iv) In some areas, the better-off actually gain more from the welfare state than the working class, for example in education.

(v) In addition, much welfare provision is geared around social control (for example, industrial misconduct), reinforcing traditional ideologies (for example, women's dependence on men), or is socially divisive (for example, the stigma associated with means-tested benefits). In addition, many reforms are at least as useful to the capitalist class as the working class; here reference would be made to the post-war 'settlement' between labour and capital which would consolidate the capitalist system.

(vi) In almost no area of welfare state provision is control in the hands of the consumers. Instead it has tended to reinforce the power of professionals and bureaucrats.

Further reading

Life on the Margins *by Alan Booth is a very informative Communist Party pamphlet on poverty in Britain in the 1980s, incorporating many of the arguments outlined above.*

Most sociology textbooks give a general introduction to Marxism.

Feminism and the position of women

Feminism can be seen as the theory and practice of putting the issue of women's subordination at the centre of political analysis and strategy. There are many varieties of feminism but all are concerned with the liberation of women from male domination. This section explores the role of 'welfare' in this process. Given the way historians and sociologists have often made women invisible, it is interesting that whilst George and Wilding (1976) point to critiques of the welfare state from the Marxist left and New Right, their analysis contains no reference to feminism and its ideological critique of welfare.

We have already seen, in the chapter on the nineteenth century, how the growth of the idea of 'the family wage' institutionalized both the reality and the ideology of women's dependence on men. We have also seen how these assumptions of female dependence were reproduced in the social insurance schemes of Lloyd George and Beveridge. Mention has also been made of campaigns by women in the inter-war years around the question of family allowances and of feminist criticisms of the Beveridge Report.

The idea that the welfare state has institutionalized inequality between women and men and reinforced traditional ideas of masculine and feminine roles is not, therefore, a new idea. Equally, the idea that women have sought to challenge this inequality and oppression is familiar also. Such struggles or campaigns occur more at certain times in history than others.

In many Western countries the period from the 1960s onwards saw a massive upsurge in demands for women's liberation. They were concerned with economic inequality, in pay and promotion prospects, with oppressive or degrading media images, and with how such private structures as the family or personal relationships can reinforce women's oppression, and with many other issues, though not initially with questions of the welfare state. The origins of this feminist revival can be linked to such factors as changes in the size and structure of families and in the labour market as well as the impact of the expansion of higher education in the 1960s on women's social and political expectations but, crucially, not on their opportunities.

114

Women and the welfare state

By the mid-1970s, feminists were becoming increasingly concerned about questions of welfare. This was partly because of their search for a theory explaining how male domination is maintained. Reference was increasingly being made to the role of the state. This led on to the way in which the welfare state's services and provision have traditionally assumed women should lead their lives as the mothers and nurturers of children and as the dependants of men. These assumptions have often excluded them from benefits or have given them benefits only if various conditions are met, primarily their conformity to dominant values about women's role in society. The strength of these ideological assumptions of dependence can be shown by the fact that they have continued into a period where the majority of women, single or married, have paid employment for most of their lives.

In this analysis of the role of the state in the oppression of women, the work of the French Marxist Althusser (1972) was drawn upon. In referring to the way the state reproduces the dominance of the capitalist class, he distinguished the repressive apparatus of the state from its ideological apparatus. In the former, he included the courts, police, and armed forces. In the latter, he especially stressed the role of the education system in transmitting dominant values. Many feminist writers have shown how schools reinforce traditional gender role behaviour. They have also pointed to the ideological role of the welfare state in reinforcing women's oppression. Thus, in the first major feminist account, *Women and the Welfare State* (1977), Wilson argued that state welfare provision cannot simply be seen as 'a good thing' where more equals good and less equals bad. She and other feminists do not oppose all state welfare, however, but they do oppose it when it is based on sexist principles.

It was not only theoretical considerations that led feminists to focus growing attention on the welfare state and social security. It was increasingly being noted that poverty was not experienced by women and men equally:

(i) Women were and are heavily concentrated among the low paid. The Equal Pay Act, coming into force in 1975, has had very little long term impact here. Average earnings for women rose to 75 per cent of men's in 1977, their highest point, and have dropped back since then.

(ii) By virtue of their earlier retirement, a legacy of Beveridge, longer life expectancy, lower pay whilst in employment, and disadvantaged position in relation to state or occupational pension provision, women form the vast majority of the elderly poor and two-thirds of the supplementary pensioners.

(iii) Women are far more likely to be single parents than men; 600,000 women are in receipt of one parent benefit (£4.55 per week from November 1985) and most are also claiming Supplementary Benefit.

(iv) Increasingly feminists have drawn attention to the question of the division of income within households and families and of husbands denying their wives and children adequate support. Because, however, the DHSS determines people's Supplementary Benefit needs or entitlement in terms of 'assessment units' based on households rather than individuals, such women cannot claim benefit in their own right.

According to the General Household Survey 1980, 13 per cent of households have a male breadwinner, a wife at home and dependent children. Of these, some will be on poverty wages and the whole family will be in poverty, even allowing for such benefits as Family Income Supplement. Most, however, will not be on poverty wages but because of the way the man distributes his income, an unknown number of women and children will be in 'invisible' poverty, not recognized by the state as being in need and receiving no benefit in their own right, except child benefit (£7 per week from November 1985).

Thus whether on low pay or no pay, in receipt of social security benefits or denied them, women's relationship to the welfare state became seen as crucial to the analysis of their economic and psychological oppression. Some of the struggles of the 1970s and 1980s illustrate the complexity of these issues.

Wages for housework

In the early 1970s some women in the Women's Liberation Movement (WLM) began to campaign for a state wage for housework. It was argued that this would reduce their dependence on men/husbands and therefore increase their personal autonomy. It would also help make one group of women less vulnerable to poverty and give official recognition to the fact that housework is real work.

The idea was discussed at the 1974 national WLM conference and rejected by the majority of those present. The main arguments against were that it would reinforce women's identification with a socially isolating role that effectively excludes them from public sources of power and involvement. State manipulation of women and family size was also feared. Some have argued that only Nazi Germany has introduced anything similar to a wage for housework and this was used to force women out of the conventional workforce into the role of breeding large families for the 'fatherland' (Gardiner 1976).

The debate has continued, however, and is at the background to many other campaigns about women's relationship to money and the welfare state.

The family allowance campaign

In 1972 the Conservative Government proposed to merge

117

child tax allowances, usually going to the man, and family allowances, going to the woman, into a new unified tax credit going to the man. This was strongly resisted by the WLM, with the Wages for Housework campaign being especially active. The TUC and the Child Poverty Action Group gave support to this resistance as well.

Whilst support for the idea of family allowance going to the mother might seem to imply a reinforcement of women's role as mothers, and carers, others argued that it would be unjust not to recognize that they did have primary responsibility for the care of children. The WLM particularly stressed the importance of family allowance as a way of providing some money to women independent of their husbands.

Eventually the tax credit scheme was dropped and the new Labour Government, apparently reluctantly, merged family allowances and child tax allowances into child benefit in 1975. This is payable to the mother. Following the 1984/85 social security reviews and the November 1985 uprating of child benefit by only 15 pence per week, many wonder whether this benefit is now under threat, not so much of abolition as of being phased out.

One feminist writer, Zoë Fairbairns (1985), has argued that child benefit going to mothers is effectively a wage for childcare. She clearly distinguishes this from housework in terms of 'skivvying for a demanding but fit husband' and argues that payment for childcare is a valid way for women to acquire financial independence from their husbands. She also argues that childcare facilities should be available for those mothers who choose not to stay at home full-time.

The cohabitation rule and disaggregation

The question of women's financial independence was at the centre of many campaigns by feminists, sometimes as members of Claimants' Unions, over the DHSS cohabitation rule. This rule states that a single woman on Supplementary Benefit, with or without children, who is deemed to be cohabiting with a man, or as it was later termed, living together as man and wife, loses her right to benefit.

The rule was objected to because it assumed and reinforced women's dependence on men and further assumed that women's heterosexual relationships are or should also be financial ones. It aroused particular hostility because of the intrusive way it was said to be enforced. Booth (1985) quotes from a DHSS guide for its own fraud investigators:

'On the first day watch the claimant's home at about the time a man might reasonably be expected to leave in the morning. If possible carry out similar observations in the evening. Watch the address again on the morning of the second day and, if the man is seen to leave, arrange a statement to be taken from the claimant. If the man's presence has not been declared, keep watch on the third day. If you do not know where he works, follow him and find out. Neighbours and others can be questioned to discover whether a man has been present, and the claimant's home and living conditions inspected to discover evidence of the presence of a man.'

Some argue that to allow single but cohabiting women to claim Supplementary Benefit in their own right but to deny this right to married women would be unfair; partly because it makes assumptions about how much money the married women gets from her husband. Thus some feminists, like the group called Rights of Women, have advocated not just the abolition of the cohabitation rule but that SB assessment units should not be the couple, the family, or the household but the individual. This disaggregation (not adding together people's needs and resources) would mean that wives or cohabiting women could claim SB in their own right. Bennett (1983) points out that governments have opposed and would oppose this, partly because of the potential for a massive increase in the number of SB claimants, possibly including the wives of wealthy husbands. Thus, she notes, feminist demands can sometimes raise awkward questions about class inequality.

119

Whilst disaggregation does not appear at all likely in the foreseeable future, there have been some moves towards greater equality between women and men in social security provision. These were imposed on Britain by a 1978 EEC ruling and a woman can now claim SB or FIS for herself and the man she lives with, so long as she is or has been the main breadwinner. Such 'role swaps' are comparatively rare. In the 1984/85 coal dispute, even after a year of being the main breadwinners, miners' wives were refused FIS because the DHSS ruled that normal earnings for the family should include the man's pre-strike wages.

Another change was in the Housewives' Non-Contributory Invalidity Pension. This was the situation where, in order to qualify for such a pension, a disabled wife (or cohabitee) had to prove she was incapable of normal household duties, as defined by the DHSS; men and single women only had to show that they were incapable of paid work to qualify for their pension. In 1984 the inequality was abolished and the Severe Disablement Allowance was introduced but with harsher qualifying regulations all round.

One major inequality awaiting a test case at the European Court is the Invalid Care Allowance. This is an allowance payble to someone who cares for a disabled person for at least 35 hours per week and who has little or no income from earnings. Married or cohabiting women do not qualify on the basis that this is their natural, unpaid function. This rule affects about 100,000 women. A preliminary ruling has supported the married woman's right to this benefit.

Further reading

There are a number of interesting and well-written books on the theme of women, inequality, and social security. Some of these are works of fiction but are excellent illustrations of the ideas and experiences referred to above.

Buchi Emecheta has written several very readable books on the experience of being a black single parent in North London. These include Second Class Citizen *(1977) and* In the Ditch *(1979).*

Pat Barker's Union Street *(1982) contains seven powerful stories of the experiences of working-class women in a Northern industrial town.*

Zoë Fairbairns has written Benefits *(1979), a grim image of life in the future, in one sense perhaps a feminist version of George Orwell's* 1984.

Another of Orwell's books has also been given a feminist re-orientation. His observation of class and poverty in the 1930s has been given a 1980s look by Beatrix Campbell (1984).

Any or all of these are worth a read, as is Elizabeth Wilson's Women and the Welfare State *(1977), a pioneer book in that area. Some of it is quite theoretical but it also has some very interesting, useful, and accessible sections.*

7

Case studies:
black people, young people,
the social security reviews

This final chapter contains two case studies of particular groups and their relationship to social security provision and discussion of the government's 1984/85 social security reviews.

Unlike the discussion of women, for example, these sections on black people and young people are not centred around a particular theoretical perspective but they do attempt to link the benefits situation of these two groups to their general position in society. Such accounts are necessary if we are to understand the full influence of social security on wider social inequalities. The section on the social security reviews is also necessary, if only because of the changes which the government is intending to base on them.

Black people

Officially there are no separate social security regulations for black people. In practice, however, the operation of immigration control and Supplementary Benefit regulations governing 'persons from abroad' often disadvantages black people in Britain, regardless of their nationality or place of birth. Before looking at these and other processes by which racism exists within the British social security system, a glance back at how issues of race and immigration have entered our account so far might be useful:

(i) Amongst the earliest forms of state response to the problem of poverty – the Poor Laws, Acts of Settlement and Vagrancy Laws – was a concern to restrict the movement of poor people or, indeed, to send them back to their village of origin. Modern immigration laws, originating around the time of World War One, incorporated these ideas and gave fewer rights of entry to foreign nationals who are poor.

(ii) In the nineteenth and twentieth centuries, supporters of welfare have, on occasion, used racist justifications for their arguments. In the late nineteenth century, Social Darwinists urged welfare provision to build a strong and competitive British race. At the same time, Chamberlain was calling for reform at home as a way of protecting the rich from revolution, and colonialism abroad to boost the nation's wealth. Rex and Tomlinson (1983) argue that the modern development of the welfare state depended partly on the exploitation by Britain of its favourable terms of trade with its colonies and former colonies.

(iii) The moral panics of the 1970s over alleged welfare abuse often used racist stereotypes to boost hostility to welfare claimants. After one massive police swoop on social security claimants suspected of fraud in Oxford in 1982, the *Sun* newspaper carried a cartoon portraying twelve of those arrested; four of those represented were black. In fact, only four out of the 283 arrested were black and two of these were not charged and a third had his case dismissed. The black/immigrant scrounger has been a frequent stereotype in so-called comedy programmes. In Rex and Tomlinson's survey a majority of whites thought blacks got better treatment at the DHSS than whites; blacks thought the reverse. Whilst the evidence supports the latter view, it does show how poverty and the social security system can be extremely divisive forces.

Activity

Using whatever multi-racial comedy programmes are currently showing, list the main ways that black people are represented. In particular, note those images or stereotypes that relate to work, unemployment, or welfare. Do you think they tend to reinforce prejudices, break them down, or neither?

With this background, we can now examine the link between race, poverty, and social security.

Race and inequality: the labour market

For the majority of the population, without significant capital, occupation or position in the labour market is the major determinant of life chances: wages, prospects of unemployment or promotion, chances of sickness and of sickness pay as well as of an occupational pension scheme, and so on.

According to the dominant ideology, merit is the main determinant of labour market position. However, much research indicates that race, gender, or class background may be better guides to a person's occupational opportunities.

There is an accumulation of evidence that discrimination systematically disadvantages black people of Afro-Caribbean and Asian backgrounds in the labour market. Through greater risks of unemployment and low wages whilst in employment, these groups are far more prone to poverty than whites. An outline of some of the findings of the Policy Studies Institute's third report, based on research in 1982, demonstrates this.

At the end of 1982, male unemployment among West Indians was twice as high as among whites and, among Asians, it was one-and-a-half times as high as whites. Female unemployment was one-and-a-half times as high among West Indians and twice as high among Asians as among whites.

In employment, black workers were much more likely to be in semi- and unskilled manual work. Black men and women were more likely to be doing shift work, normally the source of higher incomes. In practice, median earnings for black men were some £20 per week less than for white men. Women's earnings were more similar, largely due to the massive disadvantage all women experience in the labour market, black and white.

Because of higher unemployment and the different age structure of the various ethnic groups (black people are younger and more likely to be rearing children), the black population has a higher proportion of dependants to those in employment. This is called the dependency ratio. Because of lower incomes from work and a higher dependency ratio, the average member of a black household has far less money than the average white household member.

Race and social security

Patterns of claiming   As we have seen, certain social security payments are universal, child benefit or NI benefits for example, and go to people in certain general circumstances, such as old age. Others are distributed to those on low incomes on the basis of a means test. Both these principles are reflected in the distribution patterns of various social security benefits. Proportionately unemployment benefit is more important to black people, as is child benefit, whereas the overwhelming majority of old age pensioners are white. West

Indians are more likely to receive Supplementary Benefit and Family Income Supplement than whites or Asians. Given the lower wages and higher unemployment among West Indian and Asian workers, what is surprising here is not the higher rate of West Indian claiming but the low Asian rate.

Social security and passport checks The low take-up rate among Asians for many social security benefits may be related to a growing amount of research showing that black people, as immigrants or assumed immigrants, receive discrimination from the DHSS, both official and unofficial.

Douglas (1982) refers to the general principle of the SB scheme that it caters for anyone over sixteen whose needs exceed their resources, on condition that they are not in full-time work and so long as they are registered for work. Exceptions include prisoners and some patients, and married/cohabiting women still have problems in claiming.

In addition, there is now a list of others excluded: deportees, illegal immigrants, overstayers, those immigrants allowed in on condition they do not have recourse to public funds. It is important to stress that immigration rules are both new and extremely complex and people may not know that they are illegal entrants or overstayers, possibly until they make a benefit claim. It has become common practice for the DHSS to inform the Home Office of possible overstayers and so forth. This breaches the normal confidentiality between government departments and makes the DHSS an agent of immigration control.

Research by Tarpey in 1984 showed that Bengalis and Greek Cypriots in Islington often avoided claiming benefit out of anxiety over drawing attention to themselves. Many black people have come to expect that, in making a claim at the DHSS, they will be required to bring their passports, a demand only extremely rarely made of whites. This is despite half the black population having been born here and the majority of others being long term settled, with new white immigrants outnumbering black ones.

Other inequalities of treatment

Other inequalities in the benefit system include the fact that a claimant with capital abroad has this assessed for SB purposes, whereas children abroad do not qualify for child benefit. Often the children are abroad only because of Home Office delays or restrictions on allowing the family to be united.

Sometimes assumptions about Asian extended family support leads to pressure on Asian claimants to rely on their kin, despite the greater poverty in the Asian community. Gordon and Newnham (1985) claim that research carried out by the Policy Studies Institute for the DHSS shows widespread racism among DHSS staff; the report was not published.

The fact that many of the black population have relatives abroad whom they sometimes visit can give them problems in qualifying for benefits. In 1984 the time that children could live temporarily abroad without losing entitlement to child benefit was reduced from six months to eight weeks. A severely disabled person claiming an attendance allowance for a person to look after them at home or a person claiming an invalid care allowance to look after such a person has to be ordinarily resident in Britain and have been in Britain for twenty-six of the previous fifty-two weeks. A person claiming a severe disablement allowance has to have been in Britain for twenty-four of the twenty-eight weeks prior to the claim and ten of the previous twenty years. These rules effectively discriminate against black claimants or potential claimants.

Whereas many of the deprivations experienced by the black community in Britain are to do with being working class, many are specific to racial inequality. Here we have shown how a range of rules and practices put black people at a disadvantage to white in relation to social security benefits. Many talk of blacks having become second-class claimants. Problems of language can reinforce this, so that knowledge of benefits and how to claim them may be limited; in addition, DHSS interviews can be especially intimidating for someone whose first language is not English, particularly if they have no access to a supportive translator.

Activities

1 If you live in a multi-racial area, visit your local post office or DHSS office and see if notices or leaflets are printed in languages that reflect the composition of the local population.
2 Next time you see a government advertisement in the national press announcing a new or changed social security benefit, check with any papers of the ethnic minority population to see if the same advertisements are included.

Further reading

For more details on the general position of racial disadvantage in Britain, see Brown (1984); for a more detailed and technical discussion of racism in social security, see Gordon and Newnham (1985).

Young people

The question of youth

All sociological debate about youth starts from the basis that a separate period between childhood and adulthood is a social product and, indeed, a relatively modern one. It stems from the late eighteenth century when laws governing criminal behaviour and employment began, for the first time, to define such a period and when reformers, educators, and even designers began to devise special behaviour, places, and clothes for the adolescent (Musgrove 1964).

Any discussion of young people, however, has to recognize

that youth cannot be understood as a single, unified social group. Differences of class, gender, and race not only give rise to different social and economic circumstances and opportunities but different values and lifestyles as well. Such a discussion should also note how dominant perceptions of young people are often couched in terms of problem or threat. More particularly, moral panics about youth have tended to be about boys and especially working-class boys, and this has generally been reflected in (male) sociological research into youth.

This chapter does not and cannot attempt to explore the general circumstances of youth in contemporary Britain. What it aims to do is to outline how recent social policy, in terms of benefit changes, has affected young people. In doing this it hopes to illustrate some general features of the position of young people in contemporary Britain. The preceding comments should lead the reader constantly to ask how different young people – black/white; male/female; working-class/middle-class – are affected by these changes.

Young people and benefits; cuts and consequences

Much of this section is now based on an article by Janet Albeson in *DHSS in Crisis* (1985), where she combines a detailed discussion of recent benefit changes affecting young people with a valuable commentary on the ideologies underlying them.

This discussion will largely follow her division of young people into four groups; young unemployed; those on Youth Training Schemes; young workers; those studying while unemployed.

This leaves out those who remain in full-time education who will generally be either dependent on parents or in receipt of a local education authority grant. Such grants are based on parental income and may bring financial dependence on parents well beyond the usual achievement of adult independent status.

For young people staying on at school or further education college, these grants are discretionary, and given by a rapidly decreasing number of education authorities. This means that those who do not go into employment have a direct financial incentive to leave full-time education for YTS or Supplementary Benefit. The National Confederation of Parent-Teacher Associations estimates that, in 1983, 20,000 young people left school solely because of the need for money, though the General Secretary is optimistic that the Manpower Services Commission inquiry into the funding of education and training of sixteen-year-olds will recommend educational maintenance allowances for them (Hammond 1985/86).

Student grants may also be too low to prevent many students living in poverty. This poverty has not generally been seen as a social problem, mainly because it was seen as a temporary state for people whose origins were often middle-class and whose occupational destination was also. In addition, they are assumed to be single and without family responsibilities and therefore seen as a less suitable case for treatment.

(i) *The young unemployed* In 1985 over 500,000 of the unemployed were between sixteen and twenty. They have been affected by several major benefit changes. Firstly, by the abolition of Supplementary Benefit in the weeks immediately after leaving school. Instead their parents were to continue to receive child benefit for them; this transferred money from child to parent and effectively acted as an 'official prolongation of the state of childhood'.

Secondly, SB rates for people under twenty have been cut. Where their parents are on housing benefit this has been increased. This cut has increased the financial difficulties the young unemployed often have in financing adequate social interaction and lifestyles. Financial tensions and conflicts have been shown to be a significant factor in young people leaving or being evicted from home.

Thirdly, in 1985 the government introduced board and

lodging regulations limiting the time unemployed young people up to the age of twenty-six can claim such an allowance. The limitation is from two to eight weeks, depending on area. The regulations followed a press outcry over young people, especially 'Northerners' allegedly living luxuriously in 'Costa del Dole' seaside resorts. The homeless young unemployed, of whom there are 85,000, will be forced to be constantly on the move from one area to another, which will make registering to vote extremely difficult, and may even be forced to sleep rough. The policy is clearly designed to force as many young people as possible to return to and rely on their parents, though this undermines the principle, advocated by some government ministers, of seeking work by labour mobility. The legal status of these regulations, now introduced for a third time, is still in doubt after the minister's regulations have twice been declared illegal.

Finally, we should note the claim that benefit rates are too generous and a disincentive to finding work. From November 1984 the SB rate for sixteen- and seventeen-year-olds was £16.50 but the average wage for males was £61 and for females £55.70. These wages rise fairly rapidly with age but benefits do not.

(ii) *The Youth Training Scheme* Whilst the government were not able to gain acceptance for their proposal that YTS refusers be denied all SB, the scheme does mean refusers may have their benefit reduced by 40 per cent. Similarly, the government wanted the YTS allowance to be below the SB rate for sixteen-year-olds but this was successfully opposed. Nonetheless YTS rates have not risen nearly as fast as wage rates generally.

(iii) *Young workers* The government has sought to lower young people's wages, arguing that they have priced them-selves out of jobs. From January 1982, the Young Workers' Scheme paid employers to take on young workers at less than £50 per week. Research indicates that this created very few

131

new jobs; it did lower the pay of people who would have got a job anyway. The scheme has now been abolished. In 1985, the government announced that it was to eliminate wages council protection for workers under twenty-one. There are 500,000 young workers whose minimum wage levels are protected by wages councils in low paid industries.

In addition, parents on housing benefit have had their benefit reduced by £8.80 per week if they have an eighteen-year-old in work. This non-dependant's deduction is not taken off parents with mortgage tax relief; their state benefit is untouched.

(iv) *Studying while on the dole*   The government has limited the hours of study that an SB claimant can undertake. Their regulations imply a clear-cut difference between 'genuine' students and those studying while unemployed. In FE and technical colleges, the former qualify only for discretionary awards which are usually small or non-existent. Rather than provide improved grants, the government has sought to keep SB claimants off the courses that these 'genuine' students are on.

Young people and benefits: trends and comments

Overall, Albeson (1985) locates three major trends in these developments:

(i) A low priority to young people's incomes. She suggests that the cuts made by the government in benefits for young people stem from two influences. Firstly, the Conservative Government has wanted to cut overall public spending and young people are a relatively easy target. They have no major pressure group acting on their behalf, have few or no votes, and are themselves poorly organized politically. Secondly, as its New Right philosophy suggests, the government wishes to use social policy to promote its idea of what family life should be like.

(ii) An increasing delay in the recognition by the state of the adult status of young people, so that under the board and lodgings regulations the definition of young person extends to twenty-six.

Activity

Draw up a list of the ages at which young people gain various rights associated with adult status, for example part- and full-time employment and so on. Check your list with a reference such as J. Thompson (1980). Apart from their legal rights, what other factors are associated with the move from youth or young person to adult?

(iii) A tendency to transfer the support for those on benefit from the state to the family. This fits in with the ideology of the family as a single unit rather than individuals in their own rights, an ideology and a trend strongly asserted by the Conservative Government. Albeson claims that the increased financial burdens on poor families resulting from these benefit cuts can, in fact, undermine rather than reinforce family relationships.

Further reading

Apart from Albeson (1985), more detail can be gained from the CPAG journal Poverty 62 Winter 1985/86. *This and other voluntary organizations may be worth contacting. Youthaid, the Campaign for Single Homeless People, and the Low Pay Unit, in particular. Their addresses are available in the London telephone directory.*

For a wider discussion of youth, see O'Donnell (1985).

The social security reviews

On 3 April, 1984, the Secretary of State for Social Services, Norman Fowler, announced the setting up of four committees to review social security provision. These reviews must be seen as part of the New Right's aim to restructure society along more laissez-faire lines. Many of the issues raised in this section therefore are not so much new ones as illustrations of how this philosophy is being applied to social policy, even if it has been modified by opposition. A range of other general issues will also be raised and these can also be related back to recurring themes in earlier sections of the book: differing models of the welfare state, especially ideas of welfare spending as public burden; the role of agenda setting in social security debate; the question of who gains and loses from social policy changes, especially here its implications for women, the elderly, the young.

Background and agenda setting
(i) *The press*

Whilst these reviews were eventually destined to become big news, the announcement itself was not given a universal high priority in the press. Thus, whilst *The Times, Guardian*, and *Telegraph* made it their main front-page story, the *Star* failed to mention it and the *Sun* gave it the heading, 'Maggie shake-up on dole handouts!'

Two other related stories came out that day. Of these, one was about accounts of young people living in seaside resorts on the dole (see page 131); some papers gave this more coverage than the announcement of the reviews. The second concerned a research report highlighting the financial and health problems from unemployment which posed a threat to family life. This was given less priority than the Costa del Dole stories and, while the *Express* covered it, it dismissed it as 'hysterical nonsense'. The reader could usefully relate this to the account of media coverage of social security issues given by Golding and Middleton (1982), and discussed on pages 86 to 88.

(ii) *The review committees – membership and brief*

The government set the agenda of the reports, collectively the most important since Beveridge, by its selection of the committees' members and the terms of reference given to them. Including dual membership, nearly half the eighteen members were government ministers. A further four were from private industry, of whom two were in the Institute of Directors, a major pressure group of the New Right; there were no trade unionists. There was also a member of the Adam Smith Institute (see page 97) but no one from any of the major poverty organizations.

The focus of the reviews was on the cost of social security. Thus, any proposals that the committee was to come up with to change the social security system should add nothing to its cost. In relation to pensions especially, the public burden model of welfare was particularly stressed. The government's consultative document on the reviews focused on the future cost of old age pensions, especially in the 2030s – the period when the 1960s birth-rate increase will be producing peak numbers of elderly, a fact unknown in 1975 when SERPS was introduced (see page 91).

Finally, there are the issues not on the committees' agendas: the cost of tax concessions of 'the hidden welfare state' (see pages 64–5) and the low take-up rate for means-tested benefits, the general drift to which the reviews wholly endorsed (see pages 73 to 75).

Proposals and implications

The reviews themselves were not published and neither, unusually, was the evidence submitted to them. Instead the government issued a consultative Green Paper in June 1985 and a White Paper in December 1985 outlining proposed legislative changes to be introduced in 1988. The June document was welcomed by George Gale in the *Daily*

Express; praising its concern to restrict welfare spending, he said, 'At last the Welfare State is no longer sacrosanct – this reform is the kernel of the Thatcher revolution.' The December document, containing only one significant change from the Green Paper, made the following proposals:

(i) The long term value of SERPS is to be cut by up to 50 per cent. In their Green Paper, the government, true to their New Right doctrine of the minimal state, had proposed abolishing SERPS altogether and imposing compulsory private old age insurance instead. This had been opposed by a multitude of groups from the poverty lobby and women's organizations (they would be hit most by its abolition) to the Confederation of British Industry.

(ii) Family Income Supplement is to be renamed Family Credit. Instead of being paid to the woman, this will be paid through the wage packet to the, usually, male breadwinner. It therefore transfers money in families from women to men and indicates that the report's stress on the idea of self-reliance does not rule out acceptance and encouragement of women's dependence on men. (See also pages 115 to 120). It has been suggested that the minister was attracted to the scheme because of the way low paid workers in wage disputes were able to enhance their claims by displaying their wages slips. Under the new scheme their wages would look better since they would be bolstered by payments of Family Credit. It also gives employers a knowledge of their workers' other sources of income and may either reinforce pressures to low pay or act as a disincentive to claiming. Claims may also be reduced or delayed by the requirement to reclaim with every change of job.

(iii) Supplementary Benefit is to be renamed Income Support, with a variety of different levels of benefit. For instance, benefit rates for single people under twenty-five will be lower than for those over twenty-five; see page 130 for other examples of social policy acting to postpone full adult recognition for the unemployed through reduced or conditional benefit schemes for young people. There are also different rates for such groups as the elderly, single parent families and so on, suggesting to some that these rates could reflect old notions of the deserving and undeserving poor. Single and additional payments of Supplementary Benefit, for one-off emergency needs and special diet/heating costs respectively, are to be abolished.

(iv) A new discretionary social fund is to be set up to replace these two abolished benefits and meet any unmet needs from any circumstance, including the abolition of maternity and death grants. It will give either loans or grants after an examination of needs and other circumstances. DHSS offices will, for the first time, have cash limits so that, if money runs out, claimants will be turned away without knowing why; there will be no right of appeal. Many in the poverty lobby have suggested that this fund will become similar to the stigmatized charity of the Poor Law era, as operated through such organizations as the Charity Organization Society (see page 25).

(v) Housing Benefit is to be cut and all ratepayers, however poor, will have to pay 20 per cent of their rate bills. Many commentators see this as an attempt to undermine support for those, generally Labour, councils who spend more than the government wants them to, by making sure that poor people cannot vote for such councils without increasing their own rates bills.

The government's own figures estimate that 2 million will gain from these changes, mainly families with children, and 4 million will lose, mainly pensioners and childless couples on the dole.

Further reading

Apart from the (very expensive) reviews themselves, the CPAG is a valuable source of up-to-date information on this topic, especially Burying Beveridge – *the summary, by Ruth Lister (1985); or, in conjunction with the GLC,* Past Caring *(Franey 1985), a lively and illustrated look at poverty and the reviews.*

References

Abel Smith, B. and Townsend, P. (1965) *The Poor and the Poorest*. London: Bell & Hyman.

Abrams, M. and Rose, R. (1960) *Must Labour Lose?* Harmondsworth: Penguin.

Albeson, J. (1985) Seen But Not Heard: Young People. In S. Ward (ed.) *DHSS in Crisis*. London: Child Poverty Action Group.

Althusser, L. (1972) Ideology and Ideological State Apparatuses. In B. R. Cosin (ed.) *Education: Structure and Society*. Harmondsworth: Penguin.

Andreski, S. (1964) *Elements of Comparative Sociology*. London: Weidenfeld and Nicolson.

Armstrong, P., Glyn, A., and Harrison, J. (1984) *Capitalism since World War Two*. London: Fontana.

Atkinson, A. B. and Harrison, A. (1978) *Distribution of Personal Wealth in Britain*. Cambridge: Cambridge University Press. As referred to in Field (1981).

Barker, P. (1982) *Union Street*. London: Virago.

Barrat, D. (1986) *Media Sociology*. London: Tavistock.

Bell, D. (1961) *The End of Ideology*. London: Collier.

Bennett, F. (1983) The State, Welfare and Women's Dependence. In L. Segal (ed.) *What is to be Done About the Family?* Harmondsworth: Penguin.

Berger, P. (1966) *Invitation to Sociology*. Harmondsworth: Pelican.

Berle, A. A. and Means, G. C. (1932) *The Modern Corporation and Private Property*. New York: Macmillan.

Blackburn, R. (1965) The New Capitalism. In R. Blackburn and P. Anderson (eds) *Towards Socialism*. London: Fontana.

Booth, A. (1985) *Life on the Margins*. London: Communist Party.

Bosanquet, N. (1983) The Americanization of the British Labour Market. *Poverty 56*. Child Poverty Action Group.

Boyson, R. (1971) *Down with the Poor*. London: Churchill Press.

Bradshaw, J. (1985) Tried and Found Wanting: the take-up of means-tested benefits. In S. Ward (ed.) *DHSS in Crisis*. London: Child Poverty Action Group.

Brown, C. (1984) *Black and White in Britain – The Third P.S.I. Survey*. London: Heinemann/P.S.I.

Butterworth, E. and Weir, D. (1972) *Social Problems of Modern Britain*. London: Fontana.

Campbell, B. (1984) *Wigan Pier Revisited*. London: Virago.

Carr, E. H. (1964) *What is History?* Harmondsworth: Pelican.

Carson, W. G. (1971) White-collar Crime and the Enforcement of Factory Legislation. In W. G. Carson and P. Wiles (eds) *Crime and Delinquency in Britain*. Oxford: Martin Robertson.

Clarke, A. (1983) Prejudice, Ignorance and Panic: Popular Politics in a Land Fit for Scroungers. In M. Loney, D. Boswell, and J. Clarke (eds) *Social Policy and Social Welfare*. Bletchley: The Open University Press.

Coates, K. and Silburn, R. (1970) *Poverty: The Forgotten Englishmen*. Harmondsworth: Penguin.

Cockburn, C. (1977) *The Local State*. London: Pluto.

Cole, G. D. H. and Postgate, R. (1956) *The Common People*. London: Methuen.

Coote, A. and Campbell, B. (1982) *Sweet Freedom*. London: Picador.

Crosland, C. A. R. (1956) *The Future of Socialism*. London: Cape.

Davidson, R. and Lowe, R. (1981) Bureaucracy and Innovation in British Welfare Policy 1870–1945. In W. J. Mommsen (ed.) *The Emergence of the Welfare State in Britain and Germany*. London: Croom Helm.

Ditch, J. (1983) Social Policy in 'Crisis'? The Case of Northern Ireland. In M. Loney, D. Boswell, and J. Clarke (eds) *Social Policy and Social Welfare*. Bletchley: The Open University Press.

Douglas, J. (1982) Supplementary Benefit and Race. *Poverty* 51. Child Poverty Action Group.

Emecheta, B. (1977) *Second Class Citizen*. London: Fontana.

—— (1979) *In the Ditch*. London: Allison and Busby.

Evason, E. (1980) *Ends That Won't Meet*. London: Child Poverty Action Group.

Fairbairns, Z. (1985) The Cohabitation Rule – Why It Makes Sense. In C. Ungerson (ed.) *Women and Social Policy*. London: Macmillan.

—— (1979) *Benefits*. London: Virago.

Field, F. (1981) *Inequality in Britain*. London: Fontana.

—— (1982) *Poverty and Politics: The Inside Story of the Child Poverty Action Group's Campaign in the 1970s*. London: Heinemann.

Franey, R. (1983) *Poor Law: Mass Arrest of Homeless Claimants in Oxford*. London: CHAR, Child Poverty Action Group.

—— (1985) *Past Caring*. London: Greater London Council/Child Poverty Action Group.

Fraser, D. (1973) *The Evolution of the British Welfare State*. London: Macmillan/The Open University.

Galbraith, J. K. (1967) *The New Industrial State*. London: Hamish Hamilton.

—— (1970) *The Affluent Society*. Harmondsworth: Penguin.

Gamble, A. (1985) Smashing the State – Thatcher's Radical Crusade. *Marxism Today*. June.

Gardiner, J. (1976) A Case Study in Social Change: Women in Society. Unit 32 in *Reform or Revolution*. Bletchley: The Open University Press.

George, V. and Wilding, P., (1976) *Ideology and Social Welfare*. London: Routledge & Kegan Paul.

Goffman, E. (1968) *Asylums*. Harmondsworth: Penguin.

Golding, P. (1983) Rethinking Common Sense About Social Policy. In D. Bull and P. Wilding (eds) *Thatcherism and the Poor*. London: Child Poverty Action Group.

Golding, P. and Middleton, S. (1978) Why is the Press so obsessed with Welfare Scroungers? *New Society*: 26 October.

—— (1982) *Images of Welfare: Press and Public Attitudes in Poverty*. Oxford: Blackwell/Martin Robertson.

Goldthorpe, J. and Lockwood, D. (1969) *The Affluent Worker in the Class Structure*. Cambridge: Cambridge University Press.

Gordon, P. and Newnham, P. (1985) *Passport to Benefits*. London: Child Poverty Action Group/Runnymede Trust.

Gouldner, A. W. (1971) *The Coming Crisis of Western Sociology*. London: Heinemann.

Hammond, J. (1985/86) Educational Maintenance Allowances: now, not never. *Poverty* 62. London: Child Poverty Action Group.

Harrington, M. (1963) *The Other America: Poverty in the United States*. Harmondsworth: Penguin.

Harris, J. (1981) Some Aspects of Social Policy in Britain during the Second World War. In W. J. Mommsen (ed.) *The Emergence of the Welfare State in Britain and Germany*. London: Croom Helm.

Harrison, P. (1983) *Inside the Inner City*. Harmondsworth: Pelican.

Hay, J. R. (1981) The British Business Community, Social Insurance and the German Example. In W. J. Mommsen (ed.) *The Emergence of the Welfare State in Britain and Germany*. London: Croom Helm.

Hayek, F. A. (1976) *The Road to Serfdom*. London: Routledge & Kegan Paul.

Heclo, H. (1981) Towards a New Welfare State. In P. Flora and A. J. Heidenheimer (eds) *The Development of Welfare States in Europe and America*. New Brunswick, NJ: Transaction Books.

Himmelweit, S. (1983) Production Rules OK? Waged Work and the Family. In L. Segal (ed.) *What is to be Done About the Family?* Harmondsworth: Penguin.

Jones, C. and Novak, T. (1985) Welfare against the Workers – Benefits as a Political Weapon. In H. Beynon (ed.) *Digging Deeper*. London: Verso.

Joseph, K. (1976) The Case Against Equality. *Observer*: 22 August.

Kaysen, C. (1957) The Social Significance of the Modern Corporation. *American Economic Review*. 47 (May).

Kincaid, J. (1975) *Poverty and Equality in Britain*. Harmondsworth: Pelican.

Kraus, F. (1981) The Historical Development of Income Inequality in Western Europe. In P. Flora and A. J. Heidenheimer (eds) *The Development of Welfare States in Europe and America*. New Brunswick, NJ: Transaction Books.

Kudrle, R. and Marmor, T. (1981) The Development of Welfare States in North America. In P. Flora and A. J. Heidenheimer (eds) *The Development of Welfare States in Europe and America*. New Brunswick, NJ: Transaction Books.

Lewis, O. (1961) *The Children of Sanchez*. New York: Random House.

Lister, R. (1985) *Burying Beveridge – The Summary*. London: Child Poverty Action Group.

Mack, J. and Lansley, S. (1985) *Poor Britain*. London: Allen and Unwin.

McKenzie, R. T. (1976) Parties, Pressure Groups and The British Political Process. In R. Rose (ed.) *Studies in British Politics*. London: Macmillan.

Macnicol, J. (1980) *The Movement for Family Allowances 1918– 1945: A Study in Social Policy Development*. London: Heinemann.

Marris, D. and Rein, M. (1974) *Dilemmas of Social Reform*. Harmondsworth: Pelican.

Marsh, D. (1980) *The Welfare State* 2nd ed. Harlow: Longman.

Marshall, T. H. (1969) The Role of the Social Services. *Political Quarterly* 40, 1.

Means, R. (1977) Social Work and the 'Undeserving Poor'. University of Birmingham Centre for Urban and Regional Studies, Occasional Paper No. 37.

Mishra, R. (1981) *Society and Social Policy*. 2nd ed. London: Macmillan.

Murdock, G. (1975) Education, Culture and the Myth of Classlessness. In J. T. Haworth and M. A. Smith (eds) *Work and Leisure: An Interdisciplinary Study in Theory, Education and Planning*. London: Lepus Books.

Musgrove, M. (1964) *Youth and the Social Order*. London: Routledge & Kegan Paul.

Nichols, W. A. T. (1967) *Ownership, Control and Ideology*. London: George Allen & Unwin.

Novak, T. (1984) *Poverty and Social Security*. London: Pluto Press.

Nugent, N. and King, R. (1979) Ethnic Minorities, Scapegoating and the Extreme Right. In R. Miles and A. Phizaklea (eds) *Racism and Political Action in Britain*. London: Routledge & Kegan Paul.

O'Donnell, M. (1985) *Age and Generation*. London: Tavistock.

Orwell, G. (1970) *The Road to Wigan Pier*. Harmondsworth: Penguin.

Oxford Review of Economic Policy Vol. 1 No. 2. Oxford: Oxford

University Press. Referred to in the *Guardian* 22 August, 1985.

Pinker, R. (1971) *Social Theory and Social Policy*. London: Heinemann.

Piven, F. F. and Cloward, R. A. (1972) *Regulating the Poor*. London: Tavistock.

—— (1982) *The New Class War: Reagan's Attack on the Welfare State and its Consequences*. New York: Pantheon Books.

Plowden Report (1967) *Children and their Primary Schools*. London: HMSO.

Rex, J. and Tomlinson, S. (1983) *Colonial Immigrants in a British City*. London: Routledge & Kegan Paul.

Rimlinger, G. (1971) *Welfare Policy and Industrialization in Europe, America and Russia*. New York: John Wiley.

Rose, H. (1985) Securing Social Security. *New Socialist*: 25 March.

Saville, J. (1957/58) The Welfare State: an Historical Approach. *New Reasoner*; extract in E. Butterworth and R. Holman (eds) *Social Welfare in Modern Britain*. London: Fontana.

Steinbeck, J. (1951) *The Grapes of Wrath*. Harmondsworth: Penguin.

Tarpey, M. (1984) *English Speakers Only: a report of work on take-up of social security benefits with people whose first language is not English*. London: Islington People's Rights.

Tawney, R. H. (1936) *Religion and the Rise of Capitalism*. London: Murray.

Thompson, E. P. (1968) *The Making of the English Working Class*. Harmondsworth: Pelican.

Thompson, J. L. (1980) *Examining Sociology*. London: Hutchinson.

Titmuss, R. (1958) The Social Division of Welfare; and War and Social Policy. Both these are in Titmuss *Essays on the Welfare State*. London: Allen and Unwin.

Townsend, P. (1976) Area Deprivation. Policies. *New Statesman*: 6 August.

—— (1979) *Poverty in the United Kingdom*. Harmondsworth: Pelican.

—— (1981) Guerillas, subordinates and passers-by: the relationship between sociologists and social policy. *Critical Social Policy* 1: 2.

Trowler, P. (1984) *Topics in Sociology*. Slough: University Tutorial Press.

Tumin, N. W. (1953) Some Principles of Stratification: A Critical

Analysis. *American Sociological Review* 18, 4.

Ward, S. (ed.) (1985) *DHSS in Crisis*. London: Child Poverty Action Group.

Westergaard, J. and Resler, H. (1975) *Class in a Capitalist Society*. Harmondsworth: Pelican.

Wilding, P. (1983) The Promise of Thatcherism. In D. Bull and P. Wilding (eds) *Thatcherism and the Poor*. London: Child Poverty Action Group.

Wilson, E. (1977) *Women and the Welfare State*. London: Tavistock.

—— (1980) Feminism and Social Work. In M. Brake and R. Bailey (eds) *Radical Social Work and Practice*. London: Edward Arnold.

Wright Mills, C. (1970) *The Sociological Imagination*. Harmondsworth: Pelican.

Zweig, F. (1961) *The Worker in an Affluent Society*. London: Heinemann.

Index